THE ANTI-INFLAMMATORY RHEUMATOID ARTHRITIS COOKBOOK FOR SENIORS

Delightful Homemade DIY Recipes for Managing Symptoms, Reducing Joint Pain, Boosting Immunity, and Combating Osteoporosis

CAROLINE SIMMONS, MD

Copyright Page

Copyright © 2024 by Caroline Simmons, MD.

All rights reserved. No part of this book may be reproduced, stored in a retrieval system, or transmitted in any form or by any means, electronic, mechanical, photocopying, recording, or otherwise, without the prior written permission of the author, except in the case of brief quotations embodied in critical articles and reviews.

The recipes and suggestions provided in this book are for informational purposes only. The author and publisher are not responsible for any adverse effects or consequences resulting from the use of the recipes, dietary practices, or suggestions described herein. Always consult a professional or medical expert if you have any concerns regarding your dietary needs and health conditions.

Table of Contents

Copyright Page 2

Table of Contents 3

UNDERSTANDING RHEUMATOID ARTHRITIS .. 1

    Causes and Risk Factors 18

    Symptoms and Diagnosis 22

    Rheumatoid Arthritis Treatment Srategies 37

MANAGING RHEUMATOID ARTHRITIS WITH DIET 44

    How Diet Affects RA 45

    Common Dietary Triggers and Inflammatory Foods 50

    Nutritional Deficiencies and Supplementation 61

ANTI-INFLAMMATORY DIET BASICS 69

    Foods to Include in an Anti-Inflammatory Diet 71

RHEUMATOID ARTHRITIS RECIPES YOU MUST TRY! 73

DELIGHTFUL RECIPES FOR BREAKFAST 73

   Poached Eggs Caprese 73

   Eggs and Greens Breakfast Dish 75

   Breakfast Pita Pizza 77

   Caprese on Toast 79

   Mediterranean Breakfast Quinoa 80

   Eggs Florentine 82

   Chef John's Shakshuka 83

   Quinoa Breakfast Cereal 86

   Healthy Breakfast Sandwich 87

   Spinach Feta Egg Wrap 88

   Zucchini with Egg 90

   Paleo Baked Eggs in Avocado 91

   Scrumptious Breakfast Salad 93

DELIGHTFUL RECIPES FOR LUNCH 95

Bean & quinoa salad with orange 95

Wild salmon with corn & pepper salsa salad ... 97

Mexican-style stuffed peppers 99

Lemon pollock with sweet potato chips & broccoli mash 102

Spicy tuna & cottage cheese jacket 106

Rustic beans & spinach with garlic yogurt 107

Chicken wrap with sticky sweet potato, salad leaves & tomatoes 111

Tuna Niçoise protein pot 113

Curried chickpea cake with tomato sambal 114

Quinoa, squash & broccoli salad 117

Wild salmon veggie bowl 119

Ingredients 119

Steak & broccoli protein pots 121

Tuna, avocado & pea salad in Baby Gem lettuce wraps 123

Summer carrot, tarragon & white bean soup .. 124

DELIGHTFUL RECIPES FOR DINNER 127

Quinoa with Chickpeas and Tomatoes............ 127

Tuna Steaks with Melon Salsa.......................... 129

Spicy Chicken and Sweet Potato Stew 130

Fast Salmon with a Ginger Glaze 133

Kale, Quinoa, and Avocado Salad with Lemon Dijon Vinaigrette 135

Salmon Quinoa Bowl 137

Tofu Salad 141

Mediterranean Lentil Salad 143

Turmeric Pepper Shrimp Spinach Salad 144

Eggplant and Tomato Caponata 146

Almond-Crusted Salmon and Salad................ 148

Byrdhouse Marinated Tomatoes and Mushrooms 150

Indian Kale with Chickpeas 151

Roasted Veggie Buddha Bowl 153

Summer Berry Salad with Salmon 157

DELIGHTFUL RECIPES FOR SNACK 159

Flat apple & vanilla tart 159

Double ginger cookies 161

Carrot & pecan muffins 163

Smoked mackerel risotto 165

Homemade vegan bagels 167

Puff pastry pizzas 171

Sweetcorn fritters 173

Cheese-stuffed garlic dough balls with a tomato sauce dip 176

Glamorous fairy cakes 180

Easy plum jam 183

Freezer biscuits 185

Instant berry banana slush 188

Caramelised mushroom tartlets 189

Ricotta and basil pizza 192

Spiced mackerel on toast with beetroot salsa . 194

DELIGHTFUL RECIPES FOR SIDE DISH 197

Vegan kimchi 197

Gluten-free bread 201

Crunchy chopped salad 203

Easy onion bhajis 209

cauliflower rice 211

Polenta bruschetta with tapenade 212

Hasselback potatoes 215

Brown rice tabbouleh with eggs & parsley 217

Crispy Jerusalem artichokes with roasted garlic & rosemary 219

Spiced apple crisps 220

Quick pickled cucumbers 222

Air-fryer brussels sprouts 223

Malabar prawns 224

Pickled red onions 226

TO WRAP THINGS UP! 229

1

UNDERSTANDING RHEUMATOID ARTHRITIS

Rheumatoid arthritis (RA) is a chronic autoimmune disease that causes pain, swelling, stiffness, and loss of function in the joints.

A healthy immune system protects the body by attacking foreign organisms such as bacteria and viruses. However, in cases where an autoimmune disease exists, the body mistakenly attacks healthy tissue instead. In RA, the joints which are designed to absorb shock and allow smooth movement between bones, are targeted by the autoimmune process.

About 1.5 million people in the United States have rheumatoid arthritis.

The ends of your bones are covered by elastic tissue called cartilage, which supports and helps protect the joints during movements. A tissue known as synovium or synovial membrane lies next to the cartilage. The synovium produces synovial fluid, a substance that acts as a lubricant and provides nourishment to the cartilage.

In people with RA, the autoimmune process causes the synovium in certain joints to become inflamed. The tissue swells and becomes painful with every movement of the affected joints.

The uncontrollable joint inflammation can also lead to joint erosion, a loss of motion, and joint damage to many associated parts of the body. In other words, people with rheumatoid arthritis will likely experience worsening pain and stiffness, especially if this particular inflammatory arthritis isn't treated with non-steroidal anti-inflammatory medications or other standard treatment protocol.

RA affects the most important joints in the body, including joints in the:

• Hands

• Feet

• Wrists

• Elbows

• Knees

• Ankles

Over time, the affected synovium along with the cartilage and bone next to it become eroded.

Everything around the synovium meant to support the joint — muscles, ligaments, and tendons – slowly weaken. This breakdown, along with friction caused by a less functional synovial fluid leads to most of the pain commonly associated with RA.

Juvenile Rheumatoid Arthritis

This condition also is called juvenile idiopathic arthritis, or JIA. It causes swollen and stiff joints in children 16 or younger. If joint pain and stiffness last 6 weeks or longer, that may be JIA.

Idiopathic means "unknown." Experts aren't sure what causes JIA. They think some children are born with a gene that makes them more likely to get JIA. Then something – such as a virus or bacteria – sets off the immune system. Researchers don't believe it's related to allergies, food, or poor diet.

Rheumatoid arthritis is a lifelong condition. Like RA, JIA is an autoimmune condition. But kids sometimes outgrow JIA. However, it can affect bone growth, which can have longer-term consequences.

There are several types of JIA.

Oligoarthritis: This is the most common type of JIA. It affects four or more joints and usually strikes larger joints such as knees, ankles, and elbows.

Polyarthritis: When you have this type, five or more joints are affected, often on the same side of the body. About a quarter of children with JIA have this type.

Systemic: About 10% of children with JIA get this type, which affects skin and internal organs as well as joints. Symptoms can include a fever above 103 F that lasts 2 weeks or more and a rash.

Psoriatic arthritis (PsA): This type affects joints and also causes a scaly rash. The rash often appears on the eyelids, knees, belly button, and scalp or behind the ears. Wrists, ankles, fingers, and toes are some of the joints that might be affected.

Enthesitis-related: Another name for this type is spondyloarthritis. It hits areas where muscles, ligaments, and tendons attach to bone. Hips, knees, and feet are the most common spots affected, but any joint can be involved. It also can affect the digestive tract. It's more common in boys and generally starts between the ages of 8 and 15.

Undifferentiated: Doctors use this label when it's clear that at least one joint is inflamed, but other symptoms don't match up with the other types.

The Stages of RA

Rheumatoid arthritis most often develops as a progressive disease, meaning that it will become more aggressive over time. However, this isn't always the case as it can also appear in other types of progressions as well.

Monocyclic progression (sometimes called remissive) is an episode of RA with symptoms that last only 2-5 years. Monocyclic progression is usually the result of an early diagnosis and immediate aggressive treatment to ensure that the symptoms do not return.

Polycyclic progression (sometimes called intermittent) is the constant recurrence of RA symptoms and flares, but in fluctuating stages. With polycyclic progression, patients can go long periods of time without experiencing any symptoms at all, but flares usually return.

How Does Rheumatoid Arthritis Affect Your Body?

Immune system cells move from the blood into your joints and the tissue that lines them. This tissue is called the synovium. Once the cells arrive, they create inflammation. This makes your joint swell as fluid builds up inside it. Your joints become painful, swollen, and warm to the touch.

Over time, the inflammation wears down the cartilage, a cushy layer of tissue that covers the ends of your bones. As you lose cartilage, the space between your bones narrows. As time goes on, they could rub against each other or move out of place. The cells that cause inflammation also make substances that damage your bones.

The inflammation in RA can spread and affect organs and systems throughout your body, from your eyes to your heart, lungs, kidneys, blood vessels, and even your skin.

Rheumatoid arthritis in hands

In addition to swelling, pain, and stiffness, RA can affect your hands in these ways:

• A soft lump develops on the back of your hand.

• Swelling of the fingers makes them look like sausages.

• A creaking sound happens when you move your fingers.

• A clicking sound happens when you bend your finger joints.

• You can't straighten your fingers or thumb.

• The tip of your finger may be bent.

• The middle joint of your finger is bent and your fingertip is straightened too far.

Rheumatoid arthritis in feet

The most common symptoms are swelling, pain, and stiffness. Other symptoms include:

• Trouble with ramps and stairs if your ankle is affected

• Trouble walking on uneven surfaces, such as grass or gravel

• Arch collapse, making the front of your foot point out

• Bony bumps that make it hard to wear shoes

• Bunions and claw toes (toes permanently bent)

What does RA look and feel like?

RA may be most visible in your hands and feet, particularly as the disease progresses and especially if you don't currently have a treatment plan.

Swelling of fingers, wrists, knees, ankles, and toes are common. Damage to ligaments and swelling in the feet can cause a person with RA to have trouble walking.

If you don't get treatment for RA, you may develop severe deformities in your hands and feet. Deformities of the hands and fingers may cause a curved, claw-like appearance.

Your toes can also take on a claw-like look, sometimes bending upward and sometimes curling under the ball of the foot.

You may also notice ulcers, nodules, bunions, and calluses on your feet.

Lumps, called rheumatoid nodules, can appear anywhere on your body where joints are inflamed. These can range in size from very small to the size of a walnut or larger, and they can occur in clusters.

Rheumatoid Arthritis vs. Osteoarthritis

Many people confuse rheumatoid arthritis with osteoarthritis (OA) due to their similar symptoms, but the two diseases are caused by different factors.

What is Osteoarthritis?

Whereas rheumatoid arthritis is an autoimmune disease that causes joint malfunction due to inflammation, osteoarthritis is a mechanical disease brought on by the destruction of joints through wear and tear.

Osteoarthritis is the most common form of arthritis, with approximately 27 million Americans over the age of 25 having been diagnosed with it. Osteoarthritis is also most commonly seen in people middle-aged to elderly and is the top cause of disability in those age groups, though it can also appear in younger people who have sustained joint injuries.

With osteoarthritis, the cartilage, joint lining, ligaments, and bone are all affected by deterioration and inflammation. When the cartilage begins to break down due to stress or changes in the body, the surrounding bones slowly get bigger and begin to fail.

Osteoarthritis is a slowly progressing disease and occurs in the joints of the hand, spine, hips, knees, and toes. Furthermore, risk factors of this disease most often stem from lifestyle or biological causes, such as:

Obesity

Old age

Genetic recurrence or defect

Overuse of joints

Job stresses

Sports injuries

Osteoarthritis sometimes occurs alongside rheumatoid arthritis or other disease, such as gout.

Research on Rheumatoid Arthritis

In the last decade, much research has been conducted to increase our understanding of the immune system and what makes it malfunction. There have also been new therapies developed to help treat the disease. Some of the topics of intense research include:

What are the genetic factors that predispose people to develop rheumatoid arthritis?

Some white blood cells, commonly known as T cells, are important in maintaining a healthy and properly functioning immune system. However, scientists have discovered a variation—called single nucleotide polymorphism (SNP)—in a gene that controls T cells. When the SNP gene variation is present, T cells attempt to correct abnormalities in joints too quickly, causing the inflammation and tissue damage associated with RA. The discovery of SNP may help determine people's risk for getting RA and might help explain why autoimmune diseases run in families.

At conception, twins have an identical set of genes. So why would only one twin develop RA?

Twins only have identical genomes at conception. After birth, developmental and environmental factors experienced through the stages of growth differentiate the genomes. By studying the differences in the lives of twins then, scientists can better determine where and why rheumatoid arthritis begins to develop. A technique called microarray is used to examine a large number of genes at once and find differences that may develop in cases such as those involving twins. Thanks to these types of studies, researchers have been able to identify several genes that may be associated with inflammation and bone erosion seen in people with RA.

Causes and Risk Factors

Causes of Rheumatoid Arthritis

Rheumatoid arthritis is an autoimmune disorder, meaning it is caused by an anomaly in the immune system. However, doctors are not sure what causes the immune system to attack its own tissues. That being said, they have identified what likely contributes to the disease.

Genetic Factors

Certain genes may play a role in the development of RA. Since the 1970s research has shown that people with certain genetic markers are more susceptible to developing rheumatoid arthritis. The human leukocyte antigen (HLA) known as more specifically as "HLA-DRB1" was identified as a gene locus – a region or collection of genes, that is associated with RA.

Even though studies have suggested that people who have these genes could be many times more likely to develop RA than people without it, you should note that not everyone with RA has the linked HLA genes. Additionally, not everyone with the HLA gene will develop RA. These genes do not cause RA, instead they make certain patients more likely to develop it.

Environmental Factors

There are several environmental and occupational factors that, when combined with a genetic predisposition, put people at a greater risk of developing RA. Some of these factors include:

Certain bacteria and viruses

Exposure to second-hand smoke

Air pollution and exposure to certain chemicals and mineral oils

Silica mineral (found in obsidian, granite, diorite, and sandstone)

Risk Factors

Gender: Both men and women are susceptible to RA, but the disease is far more common in women. In fact, 70 percent of people diagnosed with rheumatoid arthritis are women. This may be due to a variety of factors that are involved in the development of RA. For instance, changes (such as those caused by the use of certain contraceptives) have been linked to promoting the development of RA in people who are genetically susceptible or have been exposed to a triggering event. Rheumatoid arthritis symptoms also tend to improve or disappear completely during pregnancy, with frequent flares more common after the birth. Breastfeeding can also cause RA symptoms like joint inflammation and low-grade fever to flare.

Age: RA can affect a person at any age, but it typically presents in those between the ages of 40-60. Some cases of juvenile rheumatoid arthritis do exist though, so it's important to be aware of this in the event that a minor starts experiencing RA-related symptoms. Remember: early detection is the key to successful treatment of rheumatic disease.

Family History: People who have a family history of rheumatoid arthritis may have a higher chance of developing the disease themselves.

Smoking. Cigarette smoking increases your risk of developing rheumatoid arthritis, particularly if you have a genetic predisposition for developing the disease. Smoking also appears to be associated with greater disease severity.

Excess weight: People who are overweight appear to be at a somewhat higher risk of developing rheumatoid arthritis.

Diet: High consumption of sodium, sugar (especially fructose), red meat, and iron is associated with an increased risk of developing RA.

Symptoms and Diagnosis

Rheumatoid Arthritis Symptoms

Rheumatoid arthritis is a joint inflammation disease which begins slowly and progresses over time. Unfortunately, it can sometimes be difficult to detect and diagnose RA because early symptoms are often subtle and nonspecific.

A couple of these early symptoms of the disease include fatigue, stiffness, and tenderness in the joints, which can be symptoms of other, less severe conditions as well. Furthermore, symptoms appear differently in most patients and many may have periods of time where they experience no symptoms at all.

There are many other symptoms of rheumatoid arthritis that stem from inflamed tissue in the joints. Some of the most common symptoms reported by people with rheumatoid arthritis are:

Swelling: Synovial tissue in the caps of joints becomes damaged in rheumatoid arthritis sufferers, causing the tissue to thicken and swell.

Stiffness: Inflamed joints tend to stiffen and are difficult to move correctly. People who have RA experience stiff joints, especially in the mornings or after long periods of rest. This can last for hours at a time.

Pain: Cartilage and bone within the joints will wear down over time. Joints are supported by surrounding muscles, ligaments and tendons, but, with RA, these will weaken and no longer stabilize joints. This causes intense pain and joint damage as a result.

Redness: Joints can be warm and may appear pink (or even red) on the outside during a flare or when inflamed.

The degeneration caused by RA tends to affect the smaller joints in the body first, namely the joints in the fingers, hands, and feet. The damage then spreads to other major joints in the body.

Heavy inflammation of the joints is known as a flare, and flares are common in RA sufferers, sometimes lasting for months at a time.

Additionally, RA usually affects the body symmetrically, which means the same joints on both sides of the body will show symptoms at the same time. For instance, if one wrist begins showing symptoms, the other will likely show symptoms within the near future.

RA is most common in the hands, but can happen in any joint, including knees, wrists, neck, shoulders, elbows, feet, hips, and even the jaw.

Physical Symptoms

Physical symptoms are the direct result of the high levels of inflammation that come with RA. These can affect the entire body and sometimes resemble the flu, but are chronic (or longer lasting) in nature.

Some of the most common physical symptoms include:

Fatigue

Minor fever

Loss of appetite

Skin rash

Muscle aches

Neck pain (if the RA is in the cervical spine)

Morning stiffness

Weight loss

There are similar symptoms that appear in specific locations in the body.

Shortness of breath can come from inflammation and scarring of the lungs. A sharp chest pain frequently appears as well.

Dry eyes and dry mouth can be signs of Sjögren's Syndrome, an immune disease that often accompanies rheumatoid arthritis. In Sjögren's Syndrome, the glands in your eyes and mouth that typically produce mucus and moisture no longer produce effectively.

Other eye symptoms can include burning, itchiness, discharge and impaired vision.

Rheumatoid nodules are small lumps that form under the skin over bony areas that have been eroded away. Nodules are firm and are usually non-painful. Fortunately, the frequency of nodules in RA patients dwindles every year because of early detection and symptom control. As a result, currently only approximately 20% of rheumatoid arthritis patients have developed these nodules.

Inflamed blood vessels from long-standing rheumatoid arthritis can lead to damage in nerves and skin resulting in numbness, tingling, and burning. This is called rheumatoid vasculitis.

Anemia, the decrease in production of red blood cells, is also a common symptom of rheumatoid arthritis.

Psychological Symptoms

While physical symptoms differ in severity and frequency, sometimes the person with rheumatoid arthritis feels it in other ways. In other words, RA may also cause emotional and psychological symptoms as it affects every person differently.

For example, the symptoms of RA can leave a person unable to function for long periods of time without pain. This means that jobs which involve a large amount of moving around or a large amount of time sitting still can be difficult for a person with RA.

This type of work-based limitation can lead to mental illnesses such as depression, anxiety, low self-esteem, and feelings of helplessness. All of these psychological struggles can be fairly common among RA sufferers.

If you or someone you know is experiencing these symptoms, it's important to see a doctor as soon as possible. Diagnosing RA early is necessary due to how quickly bone and cartilage damage can occur.

Diagnosing Rheumatoid Arthritis

Rheumatoid arthritis is subtle and often presents itself similarly to other arthritis diseases. Early symptoms include minor joint pain, stiffness, and fatigue, but these are often attributed to other, less problematic causes. For instance, sometimes symptoms will resemble the flu, making RA more difficult to detect.

However, people will typically feel the effects of RA in their smallest joints first, such as the fingers and toes. The earliest signs of the disease are:

• Achy joints

• Stiffness

• Formation of nodules

• Fatigue

• Unintentional weight loss

If a doctor suspects that a patient has RA, they will refer the patient to a rheumatologist for further testing. A rheumatologist is a medical professional who specializes in musculoskeletal and autoimmune diseases and is specially trained to handle the diagnosis and treatment of RA and other arthritis diseases (such as psoriatic arthritis, seronegative rheumatoid arthritis, and Felty syndrome).

Tests performed by a rheumatologist to determine whether RA exists include:

• **Family history**: A rheumatologist will first ask for the medical history of the patient to see if RA or other arthritis diseases run in their family. Many scientists believe that having a certain gene increases the chances of developing RA, and they also believe that gene can be inherited.

- **Pain history and examination of joints**: A rheumatologist can get a better understanding of disease progression if he or she knows the patient's recent and current symptoms. That's why it is so important to keep an accurate record of pain and other symptoms, to ensure a proper diagnosis is made. Once a rheumatologist understands a patient's pain history, a physical examination is performed on the joints. The physical examination can tell the rheumatologist the progression of RA and where in the body it is affecting. If RA has started to develop in the joints, a patient will often show signs or sensitivity to tenderness, swelling, warmth, and painful or limited movement.

- **Blood tests**: Blood chemistry can tell a rheumatologist a lot about inflammation levels, making it a good determinant of rheumatoid arthritis. Put another way, if certain antibodies are present in the blood, there is a high chance that the person has RA. One of these antibodies is known as Rheumatoid factor, or RF. Rheumatoid factor is a protein which attacks healthy tissues. So, if a blood test shows that rheumatoid factor is present, there is an 80% chance the patient could develop RA or another inflammatory disease. Other blood indicators include the erythrocyte sedimentation rate (ESR), tumor necrosis factor-alpha, or c-reactive protein (CRP) levels, as all of these may indicate the presence and level of inflammation in the body.

Imaging scans: Joint damage can be detected through imaging tests, making these useful tools for diagnosing rheumatoid arthritis. Rheumatologists use x¬-rays, ultrasounds, and magnetic resonance imaging scans to examine the joints and determine if RA is the cause of erosion. However, damage will not always be present with a positive RA diagnosis if the disease is in an early stage.

No single test can determine if a person has rheumatoid arthritis. Rather, rheumatologists use a combination of tests to make an accurate diagnosis. If a diagnosis is made, the patient will work with a rheumatologist to create a treatment plan that fits his or her needs and current stage of RA.

Complications and Long-term Effects

Rheumatoid arthritis increases your risk of developing:

Osteoporosis: Rheumatoid arthritis itself, along with some medications used for treating rheumatoid arthritis, can increase your risk of osteoporosis — a condition that weakens your bones and makes them more prone to fracture.

Rheumatoid nodules: These firm bumps of tissue most commonly form around pressure points, such as the elbows. However, these nodules can form anywhere in the body, including the heart and lungs.

Dry eyes and mouth: People who have rheumatoid arthritis are much more likely to develop Sjogren's syndrome, a disorder that decreases the amount of moisture in the eyes and mouth.

Infections: Rheumatoid arthritis itself and many of the medications used to combat it can impair the immune system, leading to increased infections. Protect yourself with vaccinations to prevent diseases such as influenza, pneumonia, shingles and COVID-19.

Abnormal body composition: The proportion of fat to lean mass is often higher in people who have rheumatoid arthritis, even in those who have a normal body mass index (BMI).

Carpal tunnel syndrome: If rheumatoid arthritis affects your wrists, the inflammation can compress the nerve that serves most of your hand and fingers.

Heart problems: Rheumatoid arthritis can increase your risk of hardened and blocked arteries, as well as inflammation of the sac that encloses your heart.

Lung disease: People with rheumatoid arthritis have an increased risk of inflammation and scarring of the lung tissues, which can lead to progressive shortness of breath.

Lymphoma: Rheumatoid arthritis increases the risk of lymphoma, a group of blood cancers that develop in the lymph system.

Rheumatoid Arthritis Treatment Srategies

Treatments include medications, rest, exercise, and, in some cases, surgery to correct joint damage.

Your options will depend on several things, including your age, overall health, medical history, and how severe your case is.

Rheumatoid arthritis medications

Many rheumatoid arthritis medications can ease joint pain, swelling, and inflammation. Some of these drugs prevent or slow down the disease.

Drugs that ease joint pain and stiffness include:

Anti-inflammatory painkillers like aspirin, ibuprofen, and naproxen

Pain relievers that you rub on your skin

Corticosteroids like prednisone

Pain relievers such as acetaminophen

Your doctor will typically give you strong medications called disease-modifying antirheumatic drugs (DMARDs). They work by interfering with or suppressing your immune system's attack on your joints.

Traditional DMARDs. These are often the first treatment for RA:

Hydroxychloroquine (Plaquenil), which was created to treat malaria

Leflunomide (Arava)

Methotrexate (Rheumatrex, Trexall), which was first developed to treat cancer

Sulfasalazine (Azulfidine)

Biologic response modifiers. These are lab-made versions of proteins in human genes. They're an option if your RA is more severe or if DMARDs didn't help. You might take a biologic and a DMARD together. The doctor could also give you a biosimilar. These new drugs are near-exact copies of biologics that cost less. Biologics approved for RA include:

Abatacept (Orencia)

Adalimumab (Humira), adalimumab-adaz (Hyrimoz), adalimumab-adbm (Cyltezo), adalimumab-afzb (Abrilada), adalimumab-atto (Amgevita), adalimumab-bwwd (Hadlima), and adalimumab-fkjp (Hulio)

Anakinra (Kineret)

Belimumab (Benlysta)

Certolizumab (Cimzia)

Etanercept (Enbrel), etanercept-szzs (Erelzi), and etanercept-ykro (Eticovo)

Golimumab (Simponi, Simponi Aria)

Infliximab (Remicade), nfliximab-abda (Renflexis), infliximab-axxq (Avsola), infliximab-dyyb (Inflectra), and infliximab-qbtx (Ixifi)

Rituximab (Rituxan)

Sarilumab (Kevzara)

Tocilizumab (Actemra)

Targeted synthetic DMARDs. If other drugs don't work, your doctor may want you to try this type of drug. Medications in this group include:

Baricitinib (Olumiant)

Tofacitinib (Xeljanz)

Upadacitinib (Rinvoq)

Rheumatoid arthritis Ayurvedic treatment

Ayurvedic medicine is a traditional system based on the idea that stress or imbalance in your life causes illness. It focuses on lifestyle changes and using natural substances such as herbs to improve your health. One small study found Ayurvedic treatment as effective as methotrexate, but generally, there's not much evidence that Ayurvedic medicine works for RA. The FDA warns that some Ayurvedic treatments contain metals – especially lead and mercury – that could be harmful. If you're interested in trying Ayurvedic treatment, talk to your doctor first. Very few regulations control Ayurvedic practitioners in the U.S. Always let your doctors know of any supplements you take or alternative therapies you're using.

Rheumatoid arthritis home remedies

There are some things you can try at home that might ease your RA symptoms. Research suggests treatments that might help include:

Fish oil: These supplements might ease your pain and stiffness. If you take it, you might experience nausea, indigestion, and a fishy taste in your mouth. Fish oil can interfere with some medicines, so check with your doctor first.

Plant oils: Evening primrose, borage, and black currant contain substances that might reduce your pain and morning stiffness. Some people who take them get headaches and an upset stomach. These oils also can interfere with medication and may cause liver problems. Discuss with your doctor whether plant oils might benefit you.

Tai chi: This type of exercise focuses on gentle moves, stretches, and deep breathing. There's some evidence it can improve your quality of life with RA. If you're working with a qualified teacher, tai chi is safe. But don't do any moves that hurt.

2

MANAGING RHEUMATOID ARTHRITIS WITH DIET

Rheumatoid arthritis (RA) patients require a stable, healthy diet for a number of reasons. Patients may become overwhelmed by their chronic pain and inflammation, remain undernourished, or develop medical complications

Maintaining a healthy diet is an important part of protecting your overall health, managing weight, improving energy levels, boosting your mental health and boosting your immune system. While diet alone can't treat your symptoms, the right diet for RA can certainly go a long way in helping you feel better overall.

How Diet Affects RA

Although there is no demonstrable link between diet and RA, studies have shown that the type of inflammation experienced in RA could be modulated by certain foods. Increased inflammation has been attributed to processed foods or foods cooked at higher temperatures.

It is recommended to increase consumption of foods that are considered to be anti-inflammatory, such as fruits, veggies, and cold water fish (rich in omega-3 fatty acids). As a result, inflammatory symptoms may improve and possibly lead to fewer flare-ups.

Best RA Diets

Before starting a new diet, you should consult your doctor to ensure you are making proper choices to support your over medical health. The best diets are well-balanced as we have always been taught. A healthy diet should consist of 2/3 plant-based foods including fruits, vegetables, and whole grains. Creating a proper diet for RA is no different. You should consume plenty of fruits, vegetables, whole grains while limiting lean meats and processed foods.

Below are some of the best diets to follow for helping to reduce RA inflammation and improve overall health:

Paleo Diet

Also known as the "caveman diet", the paleo diet is the most natural. Foods consumed include meat, fruit, and vegetables. Processed foods and cultivated grains are not eaten. Because this diet includes a lot of fruits and vegetables, it may be recommended as a diet for RA. However, it does also include red meat, which can possibly cause inflammation. If you're interested in the paleo diet, talk to your doctor first and make any necessary modifications.

Mediterranean Diet

The Mediterranean diet uses foods that people have historically eaten in the Mediterranean region. This diet is high in some of the foods considered to be anti-inflammatory. While it consists mainly of fruits and vegetables, the Mediterranean diet also includes lots of whole grains and extra-virgin olive oil. They also opt for more fatty fish rather than red meat for protein.

Gluten Free Diet

Celiac disease is another autoimmune disorder, which causes inflammation due to consuming gluten. Gluten is a protein found in certain grains like wheat, barley, and rye and is removed from someone's diet if they have celiac disease.

Many people with celiac disease also experience symptoms similar to RA symptoms such as sore and painful joints, fatigue, depression, and anemia. By following a gluten-free diet, many RA patients have reported a decrease in inflammation.

Because having autoimmune disorder increases the likelihood of having another, some doctors suggest being tested for celiac disease if you've already been diagnosed with RA.

Tips for RA Diet

Adhering to a specific diet like paleo, Mediterranean, or gluten-free can often be challenging and overwhelming for some patients. The most important thing in staying healthy and managing your diet for RA is to do your best at eating more of the good foods (fruits, vegetables, fish), and eliminating most of the bad foods (processed, red meats).

Here are some general tips to keep in mind for a healthy RA diet:

Try to eat mostly fruits and vegetables

Choose healthy, whole grains, beans, and lentils

Balance your diet with regular and moderate exercise

Avoid processed foods like meats or foods with chemical preservatives

Reduce consumption of refined sugars

Drink alcohol moderately

Enjoy a healthy variety of foods

If you're concerned about your diet or want to know more ways to improve your RA symptoms through healthy eating, consult your physician for support on making the best decisions for your condition.

Common Dietary Triggers and Inflammatory Foods

RA Inflammatory Foods: What Foods Should I Avoid?

For rheumatoid arthritis patients, controlling inflammation is critical in being able to live a better quality of life and improve overall health. An important way to help control inflammation is by adhering to the right diet and choosing healthy foods. Just as there are certain foods to seek out in your diet, there are also foods that should be avoided or eliminated altogether. These foods stimulate the immune system and the inflammatory process, worsening the pain, stiffness and other health complications associated with rheumatoid arthritis

Inflammatory Foods for Rheumatoid Arthritis

In addition to medication treatment plans that include non-steroidal anti-inflammatory medications (NSAIDs) and disease-modifying antirheumatic drugs (DMARDs), limiting or eliminating altogether certain foods from your diet can help you to feel better as well.

Inflammatory foods are foods that can produce or trigger inflammatory symptoms in joints and in the digestive system. These are foods that are generally processed, cooked at high temperatures, or contain lots of chemical preservatives and unnatural ingredients. Be sure to check all foods labels carefully for any of the below ingredients.

Fats and Oils

Fats and oils are very common ingredients in the average North American diet. These foods are processed and chemically altered, with various ingredients added. These foods increase the body's inflammatory response and worsening the effects of RA.

Hydrogenated Oils

Certain cooking oils like canola oil and vegetable oils are put through a process known as hydrogenation. This occurs when oils are produced by adding hydrogen atoms and effectively altering their natural state by turning them into a solid.

Many hydrogenated oils also contain a natural ingredient called omega-6 fatty acids. Omega-6 fatty acids are important for a balanced diet but too much of them, and not enough omega-3 fatty acids leads to an unbalanced diet.

Saturated Fats

Saturated fats are often referred to as unhealthy fats and they are found in processed meats and some dairy products. When saturated fats are digested they can trigger adipose or fat tissue inflammation. Try to replace foods that contain a lot of saturated fats with whole unprocessed foods.

Trans Fats

Another harmful ingredient found in processed foods is Trans fats. Trans fats help to stimulate systemic inflammation. A diet high in trans fats can potentially worsen the symptoms of rheumatoid arthritis. Any foods that are highly processed or cooked with hydrogenated oils likely contain trans fats.

Red and Processed Meats

Many meat products are produced by adding preservatives, artificial ingredients, hormones, and other additives. These are chemical ingredients that are foreign to the human body and can cause adverse and systemic inflammatory reactions in some people and in particular those people with RA.

Avoid processed meats like deli meats, bacon, and pepperoni which have been altered and cooked with hydrogenated oils and contain saturated or trans fats. Instead, choose lean cuts of meat that are labeled organic and grass-fed as opposed to grain-fed. Try to reduce your intake of red meat by swapping it for fish instead.

Dairy Products

Many people can't digest milk products due to an ingredient called casein. Look for products that include whey protein ingredients which often indicate the presence of casein. Milk is also used as an added ingredient in many baked goods like cookies, cake, crackers, bread and more.

To keep dairy products in your diet, look for low-fat options which contain less saturated fats than whole milk products and can potentially help reduce inflammation.

Sugar

Sugar is an ingredient that comes in many processed forms. Sugars called fructose and glucose are refined sugar-based ingredients that can trigger inflammation when digested. Refined sugars send out inflammatory messengers in the body called cytokines. Avoid foods like white bread, French fries, and soda.

Refined Carbohydrates

Foods like white bread, white rice, pasta, and cereals are made with white flour. White flour is a refined carbohydrate that is a staple in the North American diet. It is also a leading cause of obesity and chronic disease. Refined carbohydrates like white flour also stimulate inflammatory responses and should be avoided in a rheumatoid arthritis diet. Switch to better alternatives like corn and brown rice flour.

Artificial Sugar

When products are advertised as sugar-free, they usually contain an artificial sweetener to improve the taste. However, artificial sweeteners use an ingredient called aspartame. Aspartame is a toxic chemical that cannot be naturally processed and thus triggers an inflammatory attack response when digested.

Gluten

Ingredients like wheat, barley, and rye contain a complex of proteins known as gluten which for certain people causes an allergic and inflammatory reaction when digested. Many patients with rheumatoid arthritis also develop adverse inflammatory symptoms after consuming gluten. Gluten is found in bread, pasta and many preserved or processed foods.

MSG (Mono-sodium Glutamate)

Mono-sodium glutamate (MSG) is a flavor enhancer and preservative found in many processed foods. While there is no clear link between MSG and inflammation, it is still a chemical that isn't naturally digested by the human body. Chemical-based foods can send certain people's bodies into "attack" mode which is what causes inflammatory symptoms.

Tips for Eliminating Inflammatory Foods for Rheumatoid Arthritis

Maintaining a healthy diet can be done by simply eliminating or reducing inflammatory foods for rheumatoid arthritis. Here are some tips to help you to better avoid these kinds of foods:

Always read ingredient labels and look for indicated levels of saturated and trans fats

Compare different product brands to see which ones have lower levels of unhealthy fats and sugars

Switch to natural cooking oils like olive or avocado oil

Avoid deep fried foods or ones that have been cooked at high temperatures

Choose more low fat and trans-fat-free options when buying packaged foods

Add more omega-3 fatty acids (fish) and reduce omega-6 fatty acids (cooking oil products)

Eat as close to nature as possible by consuming less prepackaged and processed foods

If you're concerned about how inflammatory foods for rheumatoid arthritis are affecting your symptoms, talk to your doctor about dietary solutions. Remember to stick to as many fruits, vegetables and whole grains as possible to help lower your inflammation levels.

Nutritional Deficiencies and Supplementation

Malnutrition in RA Patients

Patients with RA are often at a higher risk of malnutrition for multiple reasons. First of all, weight loss is a common symptom in RA patients. It's thought to be due to the autoimmune condition itself producing inflammatory responses which cause an increase in metabolic rate. This means that the body burns through more calories than normal, which can lead to weight loss. This is not considered healthy weight loss. This type of weight loss can potentially leave the patient undernourished or malnourished.

Secondly, many patients taking the common disease-modifying antirheumatic drug (DMARD) called methotrexate, have been known to have a deficiency in certain vitamins and minerals. Many RA medications produce side effects such as stomach ulcers and other digestive concerns which can make it difficult to eat. These conditions combined with weight loss further compound the problems of malnourishment in patients. Some of the most common nutrient deficiencies in RA include a lack of the following vitamins and minerals:

Vitamin B6

Vitamin B12

Vitamin C

Vitamin D

Vitamin E

Calcium

Folic acid

Magnesium

Selenium

A proper diet for RA that is rich in these vitamins and minerals is important for keeping patients healthy.

Finally, many RA patients are at risk of developing osteoporosis, a weakening of the bones caused by a calcium or vitamin D deficiency. RA patients should be aware of this potential risk and ensure their diet accounts for this potential deficiency.

Supplements for RA

Rheumatoid Arthritis Supplements

Getting enough essential vitamins and minerals is important for your health. When you have RA, certain vitamins and minerals are even more important, such as:

Calcium

Chromium

Folate

Iron

Magnesium

Selenium

Vitamin A

Vitamins B1, B2, B3, B6, and B12

Vitamin C

Vitamin D

Vitamin E

Vitamin K

Zinc

If you can't get enough of these from your diet, your doctor might recommend taking a supplement.

Some research shows that other nonessential nutritional supplements may benefit RA:

Boron: A trace element naturally found in foods, boron has been shown to fight inflammation. Research shows that people who have high-boron diets have a very low incidence of arthritis, and there's evidence that people with RA can benefit. The best sources of boron are fresh fruits and vegetables and, depending on where you live, drinking water.

Fish oil: Just like eating fatty fish, taking a fish oil supplement can help you get omega-3 fatty acids that lower inflammation. If you're not able to get enough fish oil from your diet, your doctor may suggest a fish oil supplement.

Gamma-linolenic acid (GLA): Your body uses this omega-6 fatty acid to make anti-inflammatory agents. This is different from other omega-6 fatty acids that can actually increase inflammation. GLA is found in evening primrose oil, black currant oil, and borage oil supplements. Some research shows that taking GLA can help improve symptoms of RA.

S-adenosylmethionine (SAMe): Several studies show SAMe, a substance that occurs naturally in your body's tissues, is as effective as anti-inflammatory painkillers for relieving pain, swelling, and stiffness in the but with fewer side effects.

Turmeric: Turmeric is a root related to ginger. Turmeric contains curcumin, which has antioxidant and anti-inflammatory benefits. Several studies have found that it can help reduce pain and swelling in RA.

There are many other supplements people might use to help with RA. But there's not enough research to confirm these benefits. Medical care, medication, a healthy diet, and exercise are the best evidence-backed treatments for RA. Never use nutritional supplements as a substitute for professional medical care, and always ask your doctor before taking a new supplement to make sure it's right for you.

3
ANTI-INFLAMMATORY DIET BASICS

An anti-inflammatory diet is designed to reduce chronic inflammation, a key factor in various health conditions such as rheumatoid arthritis. By focusing on specific nutrients and foods, this diet can play a crucial role in managing and alleviating inflammation-related symptoms.

Dietary Principles

To manage inflammation, it is essential to adopt dietary principles that support overall health.

A diet centered on whole, minimally processed foods is ideal.

This includes an ample variety of fruits and vegetables, which provide antioxidants and phytochemicals that help mitigate inflammation.

Whole grains are also a cornerstone of an anti-inflammatory diet as they are high in fiber, which aids in digestion and can help reduce inflammatory markers.

Consumption of proteins should be from lean sources, including fish rich in omega-3 fatty acids, like salmon and mackerel, which are known for their anti-inflammatory properties.

In addition to fish, other healthy protein sources such as legumes (beans, lentils) and nuts and seeds are encouraged.

Olive oil, a monounsaturated fat, is recommended as the primary fat source due to its potential to reduce inflammation.

Incorporating spices like turmeric, known for its curcumin content, can further assist in reducing inflammation.

This diet minimizes the intake of processed foods, sugary beverages, and refined carbohydrates, as these can exacerbate inflammation.

Foods to Include in an Anti-Inflammatory Diet

Key Nutrients and Foods

When adhering to an anti-inflammatory diet, focus on the following key nutrients and foods:

Omega-3 fatty acids: Found in fatty fish such as salmon and sardines, as well as in flaxseeds and walnuts, these fatty acids are vital for combating inflammation.

Antioxidants: A variety of colorful fruits and vegetables like berries, broccoli, and squash provide antioxidants that protect against cellular damage.

Fiber: High-fiber foods including whole grains, fruits and vegetables, and legumes help to reduce inflammation and support a healthy gut.

Healthy fats: Utilizing olive oil for cooking and dressings can provide the healthy fats critical for managing inflammation.

Herbs and spices: Using spices like turmeric in cooking can offer anti-inflammatory benefits due to compounds like curcumin.

4
RHEUMATOID ARTHRITIS RECIPES YOU MUST TRY!

DELIGHTFUL RECIPES FOR BREAKFAST

Poached Eggs Caprese

Ingredients

1 tablespoon distilled white vinegar

2 teaspoons salt

4 eggs

2 English muffin, split

4 (1 ounce) slices mozzarella cheese

1 tomato, thickly sliced

4 teaspoons pesto

salt to taste

Directions

1. Fill a large saucepan with 2 to 3 inches of water and bring to a boil over high heat. Reduce the heat to medium-low, pour in vinegar and 2 teaspoons of salt, and keep water at a gentle simmer.
2. While waiting for water to simmer, place a slice of mozzarella cheese and a thick slice of tomato onto each English muffin half, and toast in a toaster oven until cheese softens and English muffin has toasted, about 5 minutes.

3. Crack an egg into a small bowl. Holding the bowl just above water's surface, gently slip egg into simmering water. Repeat with remaining eggs. Poach eggs until whites are firm and yolks have thickened but are not hard, 2 1/2 to 3 minutes. Remove eggs from water with a slotted spoon and dab them on a kitchen towel to remove excess water.
4. To assemble, place a poached egg on top of each English muffin. Spoon a teaspoon of pesto sauce onto each egg and sprinkle with salt to taste.

Eggs and Greens Breakfast Dish

Ingredients

1 tablespoon olive oil

2 cups stemmed and chopped rainbow chard

1 cup fresh spinach

½ cup arugula

2 cloves garlic, minced

4 eggs, beaten

½ cup shredded Cheddar cheese

salt and ground black pepper to taste

Directions

1. Heat oil in a skillet over medium-high heat. Saute chard, spinach, and arugula until tender, about 3 minutes. Add garlic; cook and stir until fragrant, about 2 minutes.
2. Mix eggs and cheese together in a bowl; pour into the chard mixture. Cover and cook until set, 5 to 7 minutes. Season with salt and pepper.

Breakfast Pita Pizza

Ingredients

4 slices bacon

¼ onion, chopped

2 tablespoons extra-virgin olive oil

4 eggs, beaten

2 tablespoons pesto

2 pita bread rounds

½ tomato, chopped

¼ cup chopped fresh mushrooms

½ cup chopped spinach

½ cup shredded Cheddar cheese

1 avocado - peeled, pitted, and sliced

Directions

1. Preheat oven to 350 degrees F (175 degrees C). Line a baking sheet with parchment paper.
2. Place bacon in a large skillet and cook over medium-high heat, turning occasionally, until evenly browned, about 10 minutes. Drain on paper towels. Cook and stir onion in the same skillet until soft and translucent, about 5 minutes. Remove and set aside. Heat olive oil in the skillet. Pour in eggs and cook, stirring occasionally, until set, 3 to 5 minutes.
3. Place pita bread on lined baking sheet. Spread pesto over pita; top with bacon, scrambled eggs, tomato, mushrooms, and spinach. Sprinkle Cheddar cheese over toppings.

4. Bake in the preheated oven until cheese has melted, about 10 minutes. Serve garnished with avocado slices.

Caprese on Toast

Ingredients

14 slices sourdough bread

2 cloves garlic, peeled

1 pound fresh mozzarella cheese, sliced 1/4-inch thick

⅓ cup fresh basil leaves

3 large tomatoes, sliced 1/4-inch thick

3 tablespoons extra-virgin olive oil

salt and ground black pepper to taste

Directions

Toast bread slices and rub one side of each slice with garlic. Place a slice of mozzarella cheese, 1 to 2 basil leaves, and a slice of tomato on each piece of toast. Drizzle with olive oil and season with salt and black pepper.

Mediterranean Breakfast Quinoa

Ingredients

¼ cup chopped raw almonds

1 teaspoon ground cinnamon

1 cup quinoa

2 cups milk

1 teaspoon sea salt

1 teaspoon vanilla extract

2 tablespoons honey

2 dried pitted dates, finely chopped

5 dried apricots, finely chopped

Directions

1. Toast the almonds in a skillet over medium heat until just golden, 3 to 5 minutes; set aside.
2. Heat the cinnamon and quinoa together in a saucepan over medium heat until warmed through. Add the milk and sea salt to the saucepan and stir; bring the mixture to a boil, reduce heat to low, place a cover on the saucepan, and allow to cook at a simmer for 15 minutes. Stir the vanilla, honey, dates, apricots, and about half the almonds into the quinoa

mixture. Top with the remaining almonds to serve.

Eggs Florentine

Ingredients

2 tablespoons butter

½ cup mushrooms, sliced

2 cloves garlic, minced

½ (10 ounce) package fresh spinach

6 large eggs, slightly beaten

salt and ground black pepper to taste

3 tablespoons cream cheese, cut into small pieces

Directions

1. Melt butter in a large skillet over medium heat; cook and stir mushrooms and garlic until garlic is fragrant, about 1 minute. Add spinach to mushroom mixture and cook until spinach is wilted, 2 to 3 minutes.
2. Stir eggs into mushroom-spinach mixture; season with salt and pepper. Cook, without stirring, until eggs start to firm; flip. Sprinkle cream cheese over egg mixture and cook until cream cheese starts to soften, about 5 minutes.

Chef John's Shakshuka

Ingredients

2 tablespoons olive oil

1 large onion, diced

½ cup sliced fresh mushrooms

1 teaspoon salt, plus more to taste

1 cup diced red bell pepper

1 jalapeño pepper, seeded and sliced

1 teaspoon cumin

½ teaspoon paprika

½ teaspoon ground turmeric

½ teaspoon freshly ground black pepper, plus more to taste

¼ teaspoon cayenne pepper

1 (28 ounce) can crushed San Marzano tomatoes, or other high-quality plum tomatoes

½ cup water, or more as needed

6 large eggs

2 tablespoons crumbled feta cheese

2 tablespoons chopped fresh parsley

Directions

1. Heat olive oil in a large, heavy skillet over medium-high heat. Add onion and mushrooms; season with salt. Cook and stir until mushrooms release all of their liquid and start to brown, about 10 minutes.

2. Add bell pepper and jalapeño pepper. Cook and stir until peppers begin to soften, about 5 minutes. Season with cumin, paprika, turmeric, black pepper, and cayenne. Cook and stir to blend the flavors, about 1 minute.

3. Stir in tomatoes and water. Reduce heat to medium. Simmer uncovered, stirring

occasionally, until vegetables are softened and sweet, 15 to 20 minutes. Add more water if sauce becomes too thick.

4. Use a large spoon to make a depression in sauce for each egg. Crack an egg into a small ramekin and slide gently into an indentation; repeat with remaining eggs. Season eggs with salt and pepper. Cover and cook until eggs reach desired doneness.
5. Top with feta cheese and parsley to serve.

Quinoa Breakfast Cereal

Ingredients

2 cups water

1 cup quinoa, rinsed

½ cup chopped dried apricots

½ cup slivered almonds

⅓ cup flax seeds

1 teaspoon ground cinnamon

½ teaspoon ground nutmeg

Directions

Combine water and quinoa in a saucepan over medium heat; bring to a boil. Reduce heat and simmer until most of the water has been absorbed, 8 to 12 minutes. Stir in apricots, almonds, flax seeds, cinnamon, and nutmeg; cook until quinoa is tender, 2 to 3 minutes more.

Healthy Breakfast Sandwich

Ingredients

¾ cup liquid egg whites

2 whole-wheat English muffins, split

½ cup baby spinach leaves

2 slices fresh tomato

Directions

1. Cook egg whites in a nonstick skillet over medium heat until opaque, about 4 minutes.
2. Toast English muffins. Divide cooked egg whites between 2 muffin bottoms. Top with spinach, 1 tomato slice, and muffin tops.

Spinach Feta Egg Wrap

Ingredients

1 large whole-wheat tortilla

1 ½ teaspoons coconut oil

1 cup chopped baby spinach leaves

1 oil-packed sun-dried tomato, chopped

2 eggs, beaten

⅓ cup feta cheese

1 tomato, diced

Directions

1. Warm tortilla in a large skillet over medium heat.
2. Melt coconut oil in a separate skillet over medium-high heat. Sauté spinach and tomato in hot oil until spinach wilts, about 1 minute. Add eggs and scramble until almost set, about 2 minutes. Sprinkle feta cheese over eggs and

continue cooking until cheese melts, about 1 minute more.
3. Transfer scrambled egg mixture to warm tortilla in the large skillet; top with diced tomato. Roll tortilla and leave in skillet long enough for wrap to hold its shape, about 30 seconds.

Zucchini with Egg

Ingredients

1 ½ tablespoons olive oil

2 large zucchini, cut into large chunks

salt and ground black pepper to taste

2 large eggs

1 teaspoon water, or as desired

Directions

1. Heat oil in a skillet over medium-high heat; saute zucchini until tender, about 10 minutes. Season zucchini with salt and black pepper.
2. Beat eggs with a fork in a bowl; add water and beat until evenly combined. Pour eggs over zucchini; cook and stir until eggs are scrambled and no longer runny, about 5 minutes. Season zucchini and eggs with salt and black pepper.

Paleo Baked Eggs in Avocado

Ingredients

2 small eggs

1 avocado, halved and pitted

2 teaspoons chopped fresh chives, or to taste

1 pinch dried parsley, or to taste

1 pinch sea salt and ground black pepper to taste

2 slices cooked bacon, crumbled

Directions

1. Preheat the oven to 425 degrees F (220 degrees C).
2. Crack eggs into a bowl, being careful to keep the yolks intact.
3. Arrange avocado halves in a baking dish, resting them along the edge so avocado won't tip over. Gently spoon 1 egg yolk into the avocado hole. Continue spooning egg white into the hole until full. Repeat with remaining egg yolk, egg white, and avocado. Season each filled avocado with chives, parsley, sea salt, and pepper.

4. Gently place baking dish in the preheated oven and bake until eggs are cooked, about 15 minutes. Sprinkle bacon over avocado.

Scrumptious Breakfast Salad

Ingredients

5 eggs

1 head romaine lettuce, chopped

2 avocados, sliced

2 large tomatoes, sliced

1 pint fresh strawberries, sliced

4 clementines, peeled and segmented

1 Spanish onion, sliced into rounds

1 ripe mango, peeled and sliced

1 Pink Lady apple, diced

1 nectarine, sliced

1 cucumber, diced

¼ cup vinaigrette salad dressing, or to taste

Directions

1. Place eggs in a saucepan and cover with water. Bring to a boil, remove from heat, and let eggs stand in hot water for 15 minutes.
2. Layer lettuce, avocados, tomatoes, strawberries, clementines, onion, mango, apple, nectarine, and cucumber in a large bowl or on individual serving plates. Drizzle vinaigrette on top.
3. Remove eggs from hot water; cool under cold running water. Peel and chop. Scatter eggs over the salad.

DELIGHTFUL RECIPES FOR LUNCH

Bean & quinoa salad with orange

Ingredients

120g quinoa

320g celery, strings removed if tough, sliced

320g frozen soya beans

2 tbsp extra virgin olive oil

3 tbsp apple cider vinegar

8 spring onions, trimmed and thinly sliced

30g flat-leaf parsley, chopped

4 tbsp chopped mint (optional)

4 small oranges, peeled and segmented

120g feta, crumbled

Directions

STEP 1

Tip the quinoa and celery into a pan and cover with plenty of water. Bring to the boil, then reduce the heat and simmer for 10 mins. Add the soya beans, bring back to the boil and cook for 7 mins more. Drain well, tip into a bowl and set aside.

STEP 2

Add the oil, vinegar and spring onions, and leave to cool slightly before stirring in the parsley and mint. Serve two portions topped with half the segmented oranges and half the feta crumbled over. Chill the remaining salad for another day, then segment the remaining oranges and crumble over the feta just before serving. Will keep chilled in an airtight container for up to three days.

Wild salmon with corn & pepper salsa salad

Ingredients

For the spicy salmon

1 garlic clove

½ tsp mild chilli powder

½ tsp ground coriander

¼ tsp ground cumin

1 lime, grated zest and juice, plus wedges to serve (optional)

2 tsp rapeseed oil

2 wild salmon fillets

For the salsa salad

1 corn on the cob, husk removed if attached

1 red onion, finely chopped

1 avocado, stoned, peeled and finely chopped

1 red pepper, deseeded and finely chopped

1 red chilli, halved, deseeded and chopped

½ pack coriander, finely chopped

Directions

STEP 1

Finely grate the garlic into a bowl for the spice rub. Boil the corn for the salsa salad for 6-8 mins until tender, then drain and cut off the kernels with a sharp knife.

STEP 2

Stir the spices, 1 tbsp lime juice and the oil into the garlic to make a spice rub, then use to coat the salmon.

STEP 3

Mix the remaining lime zest and juice into the corn and stir in all the remaining Ingredients. Heat a frying pan and cook the salmon for 2 mins each side so that it is still a little pink in the centre. Serve with the salsa salad with extra lime wedges, if you like, for squeezing over.

Mexican-style stuffed peppers

Ingredients

3 large mixed peppers, halved

oil, for drizzling

2 x 250g pouches lime & coriander rice, cooked

400g can black beans, drained and rinsed

6 Mexican-style chilli cheese slices (use regular cheddar or monterey jack, if you like)

150g fresh guacamole

Directions

STEP 1

Heat the oven to 220C/200C fan/gas 7 or preheat the air fryer to 180C for 4 mins.

STEP 2

Remove the seeds and any white pith from the peppers and arrange them, cut-side up, in a roasting tin for the oven or in the air fryer basket for the air fryer. In both cases, brush the peppers with oil and season them.

STEP 3

If using the oven, bake the peppers for 20 mins. If using the air-fryer, cook the peppers in a single layer for 8-10 mins until they are softened and starting to caramelise.

STEP 4

Combine the rice and beans.

STEP 5

For the oven method, remove the peppers from the oven and fill them with the rice mixture. Top each with a slice of cheese and bake for an additional 10-

15 mins, until the cheese has melted, and the filling is hot.

STEP 6

For the air-fryer method, remove the peppers from the air-fryer and fill them with the rice mixture. Top each with a slice of cheese and air-fry for 3 mins more, until the cheese has melted and the filling is hot.

STEP 7

Top the stuffed peppers with spoonfuls of guacamole.

Lemon pollock with sweet potato chips & broccoli mash

Ingredients

2 garlic cloves

For the chips

2 sweet potatoes (175g/6oz), scrubbed and cut into chips

2 tsp rapeseed oil, plus extra for the fish

½ tsp smoked paprika

For the fish & dressing

2 pollock fillets (about 100g/4oz each)

½ unwaxed lemon

2 tbsp extra virgin olive oil

1 ½ tsp capers, rinsed and chopped

1 tbsp chopped dill

For the broccoli mash

1 leek, chopped

4 broccoli spears (about 200g/7oz)

85g frozen peas

handful mint

Directions

STEP 1

Heat oven to 200C/180C fan/gas 6. Finely chop the garlic, put half in a bowl for the dressing and set the rest aside for the chips. Toss the sweet potatoes with the oil and spread out on a large baking sheet. Bake for 25 mins, turning halfway through.

STEP 2

Put the fish on a sheet of baking parchment on a baking sheet, brush with a little oil, then grate over the lemon zest and season with black pepper. Set aside.

STEP 3

Boil the leek for 5 mins, then add the broccoli and cook for 5 mins more. Tip in the peas for a further 2 mins. Drain, return to the pan and blitz with a stick blender to make a thick purée. Add the mint, then blitz again.

STEP 4

Meanwhile, toss the garlic and paprika with the chips and return to the oven with the fish for 10 mins. Add the olive oil to the garlic, with the capers and dill and 1 tbsp water. Serve everything together with the caper dressing spooned over the fish.

Spicy tuna & cottage cheese jacket

Ingredients

225g can tuna, drained

½ red chilli, chopped

1 spring onion, sliced

handful halved cherry tomatoes

½ small bunch coriander, chopped

1 medium-sized jacket potato

150g low-fat cottage cheese

Directions

STEP 1

Preheat the oven to 180C/Gas 4/fan oven 160C. Prick the potato several times with a fork and put it straight onto a shelf in the hottest part of the oven. Bake for approximately 1 hour, or until it is soft inside.

STEP 2

Mix tuna with chilli, spring onion, cherry tomatoes and coriander. Split jacket potato and fill with the tuna mix and cottage cheese.

Rustic beans & spinach with garlic yogurt

Ingredients

2 tbsp rapeseed oil

1 large onion, halved and sliced

170g carrots, cut into small chunks

5 garlic cloves, 3 finely sliced and 2 crushed

1 tbsp sherry vinegar

1 red pepper, deseeded and chopped

½ tsp vegetable bouillon powder, made up to 250ml with boiling water

2 rosemary sprigs

1 tbsp smoked paprika, plus a pinch to serve

150g whole cherry tomatoes

1 ½ tbsp tomato purée

400g and 210g cans butter beans, drained

2 x 120g pots bio yogurt

160g baby spinach

squeeze lemon (optional)

Directions

STEP 1

Heat the oil in a large pan and fry the onion, carrots and sliced garlic, stirring frequently for 10 mins until the veg starts to caramelise. Pour in the sherry vinegar, allowing it to sizzle in the heat, then add the pepper, bouillon, rosemary, paprika, cherry tomatoes, tomato purée and beans, and cook for 15 mins. Meanwhile, stir the yogurt and crushed garlic together.

STEP 2

Stir the spinach into the pan and cook until wilted, adding a splash of water if you need to. Add some lemon juice to taste if you like, then serve in bowls topped with a dollop of the yogurt, a pinch of paprika and a good grinding of black pepper.

Chicken wrap with sticky sweet potato, salad leaves & tomatoes

Ingredients

100g cooked sweet potato (from Lemon & garlic roast chicken, see 'goes well with')

2 multigrain wraps

200g cooked chicken, shredded (from Lemon & garlic roast chicken, see 'goes well with')

small handful salad leaves

small handful baby plum or cherry tomatoes, halved

Directions

STEP 1

Mash last night's sweet potato so that it's very smooth, then divide the mixture thinly and evenly between the wraps.

STEP 2

Divide the chicken, salad leaves and tomatoes between each wrap.

STEP 3

Fold the wrap and roll up, making sure that you contain the filling. Eat straight away or wrap in baking parchment and string (or foil) for later

Tuna Niçoise protein pot

Ingredients

1 large egg

80g green beans

1 tomato, amber or red, quartered

120g can tuna in spring water

1½ -2 tbsp French dressing

Directions

STEP 1

Boil the egg for 8-10 mins depending on if you want a soft or hard yolk, then at the same time steam the green beans for 6 mins above the pan until tender.

Cool the egg and beans under running water then carefully shell and quarter the egg. Leave to cool.

STEP 2

Tip the beans into a large packed lunch pot. Top with the tomato, tuna and quartered egg and spoon on the French dressing. Seal until ready to eat (see tip below).

Curried chickpea cake with tomato sambal

Ingredients

400g can chickpeas, drained

1 tbsp medium curry powder

1 tsp cumin seeds

2 garlic cloves, chopped

1 lemon, zested and juiced

4 eggs

3 tbsp milk

2 tbsp chopped coriander

1 red chilli, deseeded and finely chopped

1 tbsp rapeseed oil

For the sambal

1 red onion, finely chopped

2 tomatoes, chopped

10cm length cucumber, diced

1 red chilli, deseeded and finely chopped (optional)

3 tbsp chopped coriander, plus extra leaves, to serve

½ a lemon, juiced

Directions

STEP 1

Tip two thirds of the chickpeas into a bowl and add the curry powder, cumin seeds, garlic, lemon zest and juice, eggs and milk. Blitz with a hand blender until smooth, then stir in the remaining chickpeas with the coriander and chopped chilli.

STEP 2

Heat the oil in a non-stick frying pan. Tip in the curried mix, stir, then leave to cook over a low heat for 5 mins until set. Turn out onto a baking sheet lined with baking parchment, then slide back into the pan and cook on the other side for about 3 mins more.

STEP 3

Meanwhile, mix all of the sambal ingredients together. Turn the chickpea cake out onto a plate, top with the sambal and a few coriander leaves, and serve cut into wedges.

Quinoa, squash & broccoli salad

Ingredients

2 tsp rapeseed oil

1 red onion, halved and sliced

2 garlic cloves, sliced

175g frozen butternut squash chunks

140g broccoli, stalks sliced, top cut into small florets

1 tbsp fresh thyme leaf

250g pack ready-to-eat red & white quinoa

2 tbsp chopped parsley

25g dried cranberries

handful pumpkin seeds (optional)

1 tbsp balsamic vinegar

50g feta cheese, crumbled

Directions

STEP 1

Heat the oil in a wok with a lid, add the onion and garlic, and fry for 5 mins until softened, then lift from the wok with a slotted spoon. Add the squash, stir round the wok until it starts to colour, then add the broccoli. Sprinkle in 3 tbsp water and the thyme, cover the pan and steam for about 5 mins until the veg is tender.

STEP 2

Meanwhile, tip quinoa into a bowl and fluff it up. Add the parsley, cranberries, seeds (if using), cooked onion and garlic, and balsamic vinegar, and mix well. Toss through the vegetables with the feta. Will keep in the fridge for 2 days.

Wild salmon veggie bowl

Ingredients

2 carrots

1large courgette

2 cooked beetroot, diced

2 tbsp balsamic vinegar

⅓ small pack dill, chopped, plus some extra fronts (optional)

1 small red onion, finely chopped

280g poached or canned wild salmon

2 tbsp capers in vinegar, rinsed

Directions

STEP 1

Shred the carrots and courgette into long spaghetti strips with a julienne peeler or spiralizer, and pile onto two plates.

STEP 2

Stir the beetroot, balsamic vinegar, chopped dill and red onion together in a small bowl, then spoon on top of the veg. Flake over chunks of the salmon and scatter with the capers and extra dill, if you like.

Steak & broccoli protein pots

Ingredients

250g pack wholegrain rice mix with seaweed (Merchant Gourmet)

2 tbsp chopped sushi ginger

4 spring onions, the green part finely chopped, the white halved lengthways and cut into lengths

160g broccoli florets, cut into bite-sized pieces

225g lean fat-trimmed fillet steak

Directions

STEP 1

Tip the rice mix into a bowl and stir in the ginger, chopped onion greens and 4 tbsp water. Add the broccoli and the spring onion whites, but keep the onions together, on top, as you will need them in the next step. Cover with cling film, pierce with the tip of a knife and microwave for 5 mins.

STEP 2

Meanwhile heat a non-stick frying pan and sear the steak for 2 mins each side, then set aside. Take the onion whites from the bowl and add to the pan so they char a little in the meat juices while the steak rests.

STEP 3

Tip the rice mixture into 2 large packed lunch pots. Slice the steak, pile the charred onions on top and seal until you're ready to eat.

Tuna, avocado & pea salad in Baby Gem lettuce wraps

Ingredients

1 ½ tbsp low-fat natural yogurt

85g canned tuna chunks (in spring water), drained

50g cooked and cooled rice (use leftover from Prawn, butternut & mango curry dinner if made - see 'goes well with', right)

85g frozen pea, cooked, then refreshed in cold water

½ red pepper, chopped

1 avocado, stoned, peeled and cut into chunks

zest and juice 1 lime

small pack coriander, chopped

1 large Baby Gem lettuce, or other crisp lettuce, such as cos

Directions

STEP 1

Combine all the **Ingredients** except the lettuce in a bowl, season, then chill until ready to eat. Spoon the tuna mix on top of the lettuce leaves, wrap up and enjoy.

Summer carrot, tarragon & white bean soup

Ingredients

1 tbsp rapeseed oil

2 large leeks, well washed, halved lengthways and finely sliced

700g carrots, chopped

1.4l hot reduced-salt vegetable bouillon (we used Marigold)

4 garlic cloves, finely grated

2 x 400g cans cannellini beans in water

⅔ small pack tarragon, leaves roughly chopped

Directions

STEP 1

Heat the oil over a medium heat in a large pan and fry the leeks and carrots for 5 mins to soften.

STEP 2

Pour over the stock, stir in the garlic, the beans with their liquid, and three-quarters of the tarragon, then cover and simmer for 15 mins or until the veg is just tender. Stir in the remaining tarragon before serving.

DELIGHTFUL RECIPES FOR DINNER

Quinoa with Chickpeas and Tomatoes

Ingredients

1 cup quinoa

⅛ teaspoon salt

1 ¾ cups water

1 cup canned garbanzo beans (chickpeas), drained

1 tomato, chopped

1 clove garlic, minced

3 tablespoons lime juice

4 teaspoons olive oil

½ teaspoon ground cumin

1 pinch salt and pepper to taste

½ teaspoon chopped fresh parsley

Directions

1. Place the quinoa in a fine mesh strainer, and rinse under cold, running water until the water no longer foams. Bring the quinoa, salt, and water to a boil in a saucepan. Reduce heat to medium-low, cover, and simmer until the quinoa is tender, 20 to 25 minutes.
2. Once done, stir in the garbanzo beans, tomatoes, garlic, lime juice, and olive oil. Season with cumin, salt, and pepper. Sprinkle with chopped fresh parsley to serve.

Tuna Steaks with Melon Salsa

Ingredients

1 small cantaloupe, flesh removed and finely diced

½ red chile pepper, seeded and chopped

10 fresh basil leaves, cut into thin strips

2 tablespoons extra-virgin olive oil

2 tablespoons fresh lime juice

1 pinch salt

1 pinch white sugar

2 tablespoons extra-virgin olive oil

2 (5 ounce) tuna steaks

salt and ground black pepper to taste

Directions

1. Combine the cantaloupe, chile pepper, basil, 2 tablespoons olive oil, lime juice, salt, and sugar in a bowl.
2. Heat 2 tablespoons olive oil in a skillet. Season tuna steaks with salt and pepper. Cook tuna in oil for 3 minutes per side. Spoon cantaloupe mixture over each steak to serve.

Spicy Chicken and Sweet Potato Stew

Ingredients

1 teaspoon olive oil

1 onion, chopped

4 cloves garlic, minced

1 pound sweet potato, peeled and cubed

1 orange bell pepper, seeded and cubed

1 pound cooked chicken breast, cubed

1 (28 ounce) can diced tomatoes

2 cups water

1 teaspoon salt

2 tablespoons chili powder

1 teaspoon ground cumin

1 teaspoon dried oregano

1 teaspoon cocoa powder

¼ teaspoon ground cinnamon

¼ teaspoon red pepper flakes

1 ½ tablespoons all-purpose flour

2 tablespoons water

1 cup frozen corn

1 (16 ounce) can kidney beans, rinsed and drained

½ cup chopped fresh cilantro

Directions

1. Heat olive oil in a large pot over medium heat. Stir in onion and garlic; cook and stir until the onion has softened and turned translucent, about 5 minutes. Stir in sweet potato, bell pepper, chicken, tomatoes, and 2 cups of water. Season with salt, chili powder, cumin, oregano, cocoa powder, cinnamon, and red pepper flakes. Increase heat to medium-high and bring to a boil. Dissolve flour in 2 tablespoons water, and stir in to boiling stew. Reduce heat to medium-low, cover, and simmer until the potatoes are

tender but not mushy, 10 to 20 minutes. Stir the stew occasionally to keep it from sticking.
2. Once the potatoes are done, stir in corn and kidney beans. Cook a few minutes until hot, then stir in cilantro before serving.

Fast Salmon with a Ginger Glaze

Ingredients

4 (8 ounce) fresh salmon fillets

salt to taste

⅓ cup cold water

¼ cup seasoned rice vinegar

2 tablespoons brown sugar

1 tablespoon hot chile paste (such as sambal oelek)

1 tablespoon finely grated fresh ginger

4 cloves garlic, minced

1 teaspoon soy sauce

¼ cup chopped fresh basil

Directions

1. Preheat grill for medium heat and lightly oil the grate.
2. Season salmon fillets with salt.
3. Place salmon on the preheated grill; cook salmon for 6 to 8 minutes per side, or until the fish flakes easily with a fork.
4. Combine water, rice vinegar, brown sugar, chile paste, ginger, garlic, and soy sauce in a small saucepan over medium heat.

5. Bring mixture to a boil, reduce heat to medium and simmer until barely thickened, about 2 minutes.
6. Sprinkle basil on top of salmon; spoon glaze over basil.

Kale, Quinoa, and Avocado Salad with Lemon Dijon Vinaigrette

Ingredients

Salad

⅔ cup quinoa

1 ⅓ cups water

1 bunch kale, torn into bite-sized pieces

½ avocado - peeled, pitted, and diced

½ cup chopped cucumber

⅓ cup chopped red bell pepper

2 tablespoons chopped red onion

1 tablespoon crumbled feta cheese

Dressing

¼ cup olive oil

2 tablespoons lemon juice

1 ½ tablespoons Dijon mustard

¾ teaspoon sea salt

¼ teaspoon ground black pepper

Directions

1. Bring the quinoa and 1 1/3 cup water to a boil in a saucepan. Reduce heat to medium-low, cover,

and simmer until the quinoa is tender, and the water has been absorbed, about 15 to 20 minutes. Set aside to cool.

2. Place kale in a steamer basket over 1 inch of boiling water in a saucepan. Cover saucepan with a lid and steam kale until hot, about 45 seconds; transfer to a large plate. Top kale with quinoa, avocado, cucumber, bell pepper, red onion, and feta cheese.
3. Whisk olive oil, lemon juice, Dijon mustard, sea salt, and black pepper together in a bowl until the oil emulsifies into the dressing; pour over the salad.

Salmon Quinoa Bowl

Ingredients

1 cup white quinoa

1 ¾ cups water

Dressing:

½ cup Greek yogurt

¼ cup tahini

1 tablespoon lemon juice

½ teaspoon grated garlic

3 tablespoons water, or as needed

½ teaspoon kosher salt

Salad:

1 ½ (8 ounce) packages lacinato kale

2 carrots

2 (15 ounce) cans chickpeas, drained and rinsed

½ cup dried cherries

1 tablespoon olive oil

4 (4 ounce) skin-on salmon fillets

Directions

1. Stir together quinoa and water in a medium saucepan over medium-high heat; bring to a boil. Reduce heat to medium-low, cover, and cook until tender, about 12 minutes. Remove from heat and keep covered; let sit for 3 to 5 minutes. Set aside.
2. Stir together yogurt, tahini, lemon juice, and garlic in a large bowl for the salad. Add water, 1 tablespoon at a time, until desired consistency is reached. Season with salt. Set aside.
3. Pull stems off the kale. Tear the leaves and place in the bowl with the dressing. Shave carrots into long ribbons and add to the bowl. Massage

dressing into the salad until fully coated, about 1 minute. Add chickpeas and cherries to kale; toss to coat.

4. Heat oil in a large nonstick skillet over medium heat. Cook salmon, skin-side-down, until crisp, about 4 minutes. Flip and cook until desired degree of doneness is reached, 3 to 4 minutes more for medium rare. Remove to a plate.

5. Divide quinoa between 4 bowls. Add the kale salad and top with salmon. Top with a drizzle of olive oil, crack in some black pepper, and serve immediately.

Cook's Note:

You can easily substitute Greek yogurt with some avocado for a dairy-free option.

Tofu Salad

Ingredients

Marinated Tofu:

1 tablespoon sweet chili sauce

1 tablespoon dark soy sauce

1 tablespoon sesame oil

2 cloves garlic, crushed

½ teaspoon grated fresh ginger root

8 ounces extra-firm tofu, drained and diced

Salad:

1 cup snow peas, trimmed

1 cup finely shredded red cabbage

2 small carrots, grated

2 tablespoons chopped peanuts

Directions

1. Make the tofu: Whisk chili sauce, soy sauce, sesame oil, garlic, and ginger together in a large bowl. Add tofu and toss to coat. Cover and marinate for 1 hour in the refrigerator.
2. When the tofu is almost finished marinating, bring a pot of water to a boil. Add snow peas and blanch for 1 to 2 minutes. Transfer with a slotted spoon to a bowl of cold water. Drain and blot dry.
3. Make the salad: Combine snow peas, cabbage, carrots, and peanuts in a bowl. Add tofu and marinade and toss gently to combine.

Mediterranean Lentil Salad

Ingredients

1 cup dry brown lentils

1 cup diced carrots

1 cup red onion, diced

2 cloves garlic, minced

1 bay leaf

½ teaspoon dried thyme

2 tablespoons lemon juice

½ cup diced celery

¼ cup chopped parsley

1 teaspoon salt

¼ teaspoon ground black pepper

¼ cup olive oil

Directions

1. Combine lentils, carrots, onion, garlic, bay leaf, and thyme in a saucepan. Add enough water to cover by 1 inch; bring to a boil, reduce heat and simmer uncovered for 15 to 20 minutes or until lentils are tender but not mushy.
2. Drain lentils and vegetables and remove bay leaf. Add olive oil, lemon juice, celery, parsley, salt and pepper. Toss gently to mix and serve at room temperature.

Turmeric Pepper Shrimp Spinach Salad

Ingredients

1 teaspoon ghee (clarified butter)

7 prawns, peeled and deveined

¼ teaspoon ground turmeric

¼ teaspoon freshly ground black pepper

1 cup fresh baby spinach, or to taste

½ avocado - peeled, pitted, and sliced

½ apple - peeled, cored, and thinly sliced

2 tablespoons crumbled feta cheese

1 tablespoon sliced almonds, or to taste

1 tablespoon extra-virgin olive oil

1 pinch Himalayan pink salt to taste

Directions

1. Heat a small skillet over medium heat; add ghee. Place prawns in the melted ghee and season with

turmeric and pepper; cook for 30 seconds. Flip prawns and cook other side until pink and cooked through, 30 to 60 seconds. Remove skillet from heat.

2. Place spinach in a bowl and top with avocado, apple slices, and shrimp. Sprinkle feta cheese and almonds over salad. Drizzle olive oil over salad and top with salt.

Eggplant and Tomato Caponata

Ingredients

1 tablespoon olive oil

2 Japanese eggplant, cut into 1/2-inch cubes

1 yellow onion, chopped

3 cloves garlic, minced

1 (14.5 ounce) can fire-roasted tomatoes (such as Hunt's®)

⅓ cup red wine

1 ½ tablespoons capers

2 teaspoons dried oregano

1 teaspoon ground cinnamon

1 teaspoon ground allspice

1 teaspoon unsweetened cocoa powder

½ teaspoon white sugar

1 bay leaf

Directions

1. Heat olive oil in a skillet over medium-high heat; saute eggplant, onion, and garlic until lightly

browned, 5 to 7 minutes. Add tomatoes, red wine, and capers and simmer until heated through, about 5 minutes.

2. Mix oregano, cinnamon, allspice, cocoa powder, sugar, and bay leaf into eggplant mixture; simmer until thickened, 30 minutes. Add a few tablespoons water if mixture becomes too thick. Remove bay leaf.

Almond-Crusted Salmon and Salad

Ingredients

2 tablespoons olive oil, divided

2 teaspoons lemon juice, divided

salt and ground black pepper to taste

2 (8 ounce) fillets wild salmon fillets

½ teaspoon Himalayan salt, or to taste

½ cup finely crushed almonds

1 (6 ounce) package baby spinach leaves

1 cup cherry tomatoes

Directions

1. Preheat the oven to 500 degrees F (260 degrees C). Grease a baking pan with 1 tablespoon olive oil.
2. Mix remaining olive oil, 1 teaspoon lemon juice, salt, and black pepper together in a bowl to form the salad dressing.
3. Brush salmon fillets with remaining 1 teaspoon lemon juice. Sprinkle with Himalayan salt and black pepper. Cover top and sides of salmon with almonds. Place salmon skin-side down in the prepared baking pan. Sprinkle any

remaining almonds on top, pressing gently to adhere.
4. Bake in the preheated oven until salmon flakes easily with a fork, about 15 minutes. Let cool; cut each fillet in half.
5. Place spinach and tomatoes in a bowl. Add dressing; toss to coat. Serve alongside the salmon.

Byrdhouse Marinated Tomatoes and Mushrooms

Ingredients

¼ cup balsamic vinegar

⅓ cup vegetable oil

1 ½ teaspoons white sugar

½ teaspoon salt

½ teaspoon ground black pepper

12 ounces cherry tomatoes, halved

1 (8 ounce) package fresh mushrooms

2 green onions, sliced

½ cup chopped fresh basil

Directions

Whisk together the balsamic vinegar, vegetable oil, sugar, salt, and pepper in a bowl; add the tomatoes, mushrooms, onions, and basil; toss until evenly coated. Cover and chill in refrigerator at least 3 hours. Stir before serving.

Indian Kale with Chickpeas

Ingredients

2 tablespoons olive oil, or as needed

1 onion, finely chopped

1 red chile pepper, seeded and sliced

1 (14 ounce) can chickpeas, drained

1 tablespoon ground cumin

1 teaspoon ground coriander

½ teaspoon ground turmeric

1 pinch ground cinnamon

1 pinch sea salt

1 lemon, zested and juiced

1 cup roughly chopped kale, or more to taste

Directions

1. Heat oil in a large frying pan or wok over medium-high heat. Add onion and chile pepper; saute until onion is tender, 5 to 7 minutes. Add chickpeas, cumin, coriander, turmeric, cinnamon, and salt; saute for 5 minutes. Pour in a splash of water, followed by lemon zest and juice. Season further to taste if desired.
2. Fold kale into the mixture until just wilted, 3 to 5 minutes. Remove from heat and serve.

Roasted Veggie Buddha Bowl

Ingredients

1 cup water

½ cup bulgur

1 sweet potato, peeled and cut into 1-inch cubes

4 teaspoons olive oil, divided

salt and ground black pepper to taste

½ pound fennel bulb, trimmed and cut into 1-inch cubes

1 small red onion, cut into 1-inch pieces

1 red bell pepper, cut into 1-inch strips

1 (8 ounce) package tempeh, cut into 1-inch pieces

½ teaspoon curry powder

2 teaspoons coconut oil

Orange-Curry Dressing:

¼ cup fresh squeezed orange juice

2 tablespoons olive oil

2 teaspoons red wine vinegar

½ teaspoon curry powder

¼ teaspoon salt

¼ teaspoon ground black pepper

2 tablespoons raw pumpkin seeds (pepitas)

Directions

1. Preheat oven to 400 degrees F (200 degrees C). Line a baking sheet with parchment paper.
2. Bring water and bulgur to a boil in a saucepan; cover and reduce heat to medium-low. Simmer until water is absorbed and bulgur is soft, about 12 minutes. Keep warm.
3. Place sweet potato in a bowl and drizzle 1 teaspoon olive oil over it; season with salt and pepper. Toss to coat. Transfer sweet potato to the prepared baking sheet, placing in 1 row. Place fennel in the same bowl, add 1 teaspoon olive oil, and season with salt and pepper. Toss

to coat and place fennel next to sweet potato, keeping each separate.

4. Roast in the preheated oven for 10 minutes. Place red onion in the same bowl; add 1 teaspoon olive oil, and season with salt and pepper. Toss to coat and place on the baking sheet with sweet potato and fennel, keeping them separate. Place red bell pepper in the same bowl; add 1 teaspoon olive oil, and season with salt and pepper. Toss to coat and place on the baking sheet next to the onion.

5. Roast in the oven until all the vegetables are cooked to desired doneness, 10 to 15 minutes.

6. Place tempeh in a bowl and season with 1/2 teaspoon curry powder, tossing to coat.

7. Heat coconut oil in a skillet over medium-high heat; saute tempeh, turning occasionally, until all sides are evenly browned, about 10 minutes.

8. Whisk orange juice, 2 tablespoons olive oil, red wine vinegar, 1/2 teaspoon curry powder, 1/4 teaspoon salt, and 1/4 teaspoon pepper in a small bowl until dressing is smooth.
9. Divide bulgur between 2 bowls. Place half of sweet potato, fennel, red onion, and red bell pepper around bulgur; top each with 1 tablespoon pumpkin seeds. Drizzle dressing over each bowl.

Summer Berry Salad with Salmon

Ingredients

8 cups washed and chopped green leaf lettuce

12 ounces cooked and chilled salmon, flaked into bite-sized chunks

1 cup fresh blackberries

1 cup fresh raspberries

1 cup sliced fresh strawberries

⅓ cup honey mustard dressing

Directions

1. Combine lettuce, salmon, blackberries, raspberries, and strawberries in a large bowl and toss gently to combine.
2. Drizzle salad with dressing and toss gently to coat.

DELIGHTFUL RECIPES FOR SNACK

Flat apple & vanilla tart

Ingredients

375g pack puff pastry, preferably all-butter

5 large eating apples - Cox's, russets or Elstar

juice of 1 lemon

25g butter, cut into small pieces

3 tsp vanilla sugar or 1 tsp vanilla extract

1 tbsp caster sugar

3 rounded tbsp apricot conserve

Directions

STEP 1

Heat oven to 220C/fan 200C/gas 7. Roll out the pastry and trim to a round about 35cm across. Transfer to a baking sheet lined with parchment paper.

STEP 2

Peel, core and thinly slice the apples and toss in the lemon juice. Spread over the pastry to within 2cm of the edges. Curl up the edges slightly to stop the juices running off.

STEP 3

Dot the top with the butter and sprinkle with vanilla and caster sugar. Bake for 15-20 mins until the apples are tender and the pastry crisp.

STEP 4

Warm the conserve and brush over the apples and pastry edge. Serve hot with vanilla ice cream or crème fraîche.

Double ginger cookies

Ingredients

350g plain flour

1 tbsp ground ginger

1 tsp bicarbonate of soda

175g light muscovado sugar

100g butter, chopped

8 pieces of stem ginger, chopped (not too finely), plus thin slices, to decorate (optional)

1 large egg

4 tbsp golden syrup

200g bar dark chocolate, chopped

Directions

STEP 1

Mix the flour, ground ginger, bicarbonate of soda, 1/2 tsp salt and sugar in a bowl, then rub in the butter to make crumbs. Stir in the chopped stem ginger.

STEP 2

Beat together the egg and syrup, pour into the dry Ingredients and stir, then knead with your hands to make a dough. Cut the dough in half and shape each piece into a thick sausage about 6cm across, making sure that the ends are straight. Wrap in cling film and chill for 20 mins. You can now freeze all or part of the dough for 2 months.

Carrot & pecan muffins

Ingredients

2 x 400g can cannellini beans in water, drained

2 tsp ground cinnamon

100g porridge oats

4 large eggs

2 tbsp rapeseed oil

4 tbsp maple syrup

2 tsp vanilla extract

zest 1 large orange

170g carrot, coarsely grated

100g raisins

80g pecan halves, 12 reserved, the rest roughly chopped

2 tsp baking powder

Directions

STEP 1

Heat oven to 180C/160C fan/gas 4 and line a 12-hole muffin tin with paper cases. Tip the beans into a bowl and add the cinnamon, oats, eggs, oil, maple syrup, vanilla extract and orange zest. Blitz with a hand blender until really smooth – the beans and oats should be ground down as much as possible.

STEP 2

Stir in the carrot, raisins, chopped pecans and baking powder, and mix well. Spoon into the muffin cases – use a large ice cream scoop if you have one, to get nice even muffins.

STEP 3

Top each muffin with a reserved pecan and bake for 20 mins until set and light brown. Cool on a wire rack. Will keep in the fridge for a few days, or freeze for 6 weeks; thaw at room temperature.

Smoked mackerel risotto

Ingredients

1 tbsp butter

1 onion, finely chopped

250g risotto rice

100ml white wine

1l vegetable stock

1 x 240 pack smoked mackerel

2 spring onions, sliced

100g bag fresh spinach

Directions

STEP 1

Heat the butter in a large frying pan. Tip in the onion, then fry gently for 5 mins until softened. Stir in the rice and mix until coated in the butter, then pour in the wine and let it bubble until it's almost all disappeared.

STEP 2

Pour in half the stock, give it a good stir, then leave to gently cook for 10 mins. Add half of the remaining stock, stir again and cook for 5 mins more. Keep adding stock and cooking until the rice is tender.

STEP 3

Peel the skin off the mackerel, scrape away any dark brown flesh, then flake. Stir into the rice with the spring onions and spinach, then cook just until the spinach has wilted slightly. Serve straight away.

Homemade vegan bagels

Ingredients

7g sachet dried yeast

4 tbsp sugar

2 tsp salt

450g bread flour

poppy, fennel and/or sesame seeds to sprinkle on top (optional)

Directions

STEP 1

Tip the yeast and 1 tbsp sugar into a large bowl, and pour over 100ml warm water. Leave for 10 mins until the mixture becomes frothy.

STEP 2

Pour 200ml warm water into the bowl, then stir in the salt and half the flour. Keep adding the remaining flour (you may not have to use it all) and mixing with your hands until you have a soft but not sticky dough. Then knead for 10 mins until the dough feels smooth and elastic. Shape into a ball and put in a clean, lightly oiled bowl. Cover loosely and leave in a warm place until doubled in size, about 1hr.

STEP 3

Heat the oven to 220C/200C fan/gas 7. On a lightly floured surface, divide the dough into 10 pieces, each about 85g. Shape each piece into a flattish ball, then take a wooden spoon and use the handle to make a hole in the middle of each ball. Slip the spoon into the hole, then twirl the bagel around the spoon to make a hole about 3cm wide. Cover the bagel loosely while you shape the remaining dough.

STEP 4

Meanwhile, bring a large pan of water to the boil and tip in the remaining sugar. Slip the bagels into the boiling water – no more than four at a time. Cook for 1-2 mins, turning over in the water until the bagels have puffed slightly and a skin has formed. Remove with a slotted spoon and drain away any excess water. Sprinkle over your choice of topping and place on a baking tray lined with parchment. Bake in the oven for 25 mins until browned and crisp – the bases should sound hollow when tapped. Leave to cool on a wire rack, then serve with your favourite filling.

Puff pastry pizzas

Ingredients

320g sheet ready-rolled light puff pastry

6 tbsp tomato purée

1 tbsp tomato ketchup

1 tsp dried oregano

75g mozzarella or cheddar

For the topping

sweetcorn, olives, peppers, red onion, cherry tomatoes, spinach, basil

Directions

STEP 1

Heat the oven to 200C/180C fan/gas 6, or if using an air-fryer, heat it to 180C for 4 mins. Unroll the pastry, cut into six squares and arrange over two baking trays lined with baking parchment. Use a cutlery knife to score a 1cm border around the edge of each pastry square. Bake in the oven for 15 mins, until puffed up but not cooked through. Or, if using an air-fryer, bake the batch for 8 mins. You might need to do this in two batches.

STEP 2

While the pastry cooks, make the sauce and prepare your toppings. Mix the tomato purée, tomato ketchup, oregano and 1 tbsp water. Grate the cheese and chop any veg or herbs you want to put on top into small pieces. Set aside.

STEP 3

Remove the pastry from the oven or air-fryer and squash down the middles with the back of a spoon. Divide the sauce between the pastry squares and spread it out to the puffed-up edges. Sprinkle with the cheese, then add your toppings. Bake for another 5-8 mins in the oven or 5 mins in the air-fryer and serve.

Sweetcorn fritters

Ingredients

150g self-raising flour

1 tsp baking powder

1 tsp smoked paprika

160ml whole milk

1 egg

550g sweetcorn

2 spring onions, chopped, plus a little extra cut into thin strips to serve (optional)

10g sliced chives

handful of parsley, chopped

rapeseed oil, for frying

Directions

STEP 1

Mix the flour, baking powder, paprika and milk together in a large bowl. Mix in the egg, followed by the sweetcorn, chopped spring onions, chives, parsley, 1 tsp salt and some freshly ground black pepper.

STEP 2

Heat a 1cm depth of oil in a frying pan over a medium heat until a small amount of the fritter mixture sizzles when dropped in. For larger fritters, drop 2 heaped tablespoons of the mixture into the pan at a time in a clockwise direction (this will help you remember the order they were added to the pan, so you can flip them at the right stage). For smaller fritters, do the same, but with 1 heaped tablespoon of mixture at a time.

STEP 3

After 2 mins, flip the fritters over in the same order they were added to the pan. Cook for another 2 mins, continuing to turn every now and then to ensure both sides are evenly golden brown. When ready, the fritters should be darker brown with crispy pieces of corn at the edges – be careful, as some of the kernels may burst during the cooking process. Remove to a wire rack and pat away any excess oil using kitchen paper. Serve straightaway with a few strips of spring onion scattered over, if you like.

Cheese-stuffed garlic dough balls with a tomato sauce dip

Ingredients

50g butter, cubed

300g strong white bread flour

7g sachet fast-action dried yeast

1 tbsp caster sugar

200g block mozzarella, cut into 1.5cm cubes

65g gruyère, coarsely grated (optional)

For the garlic butter

100g butter

2 garlic cloves, crushed

1 rosemary sprig, leaves picked and finely chopped

For the tomato sauce dip

1 tbsp olive oil, plus extra for the bowl and baking sheet

1 garlic clove, sliced

250g passata

1 tsp red wine vinegar

1 tsp caster sugar

pinch of chilli flakes

½ small bunch of basil, torn, plus extra to serve

Directions

STEP 1

Heat 175ml water in a saucepan until steaming, then add the butter. Remove from the heat and leave to cool until the mixture is just warm (it should not be hot). Combine the flour, yeast, sugar and 1 tsp salt in a large bowl or stand mixer. Add the cooled butter mixture, and mix to a soft dough using a wooden spoon or the mixer. Knead for 10 mins by hand (or 5 mins using a mixer) until the dough feels bouncy and smooth. Transfer to an oiled bowl and cover with a clean tea towel. Leave somewhere warm to rise for 1½-2 hrs, or until doubled in size. Alternatively, leave to prove in the fridge overnight.

STEP 2

Oil and line a baking sheet with baking parchment. Knock the air out of the dough, then knead again for several minutes. Flatten a small piece of dough (about 20g) into a disc, and put a cube of the mozzarella and a pinch of the gruyère into the middle of the disc. Enclose the cheeses with the dough, then roll into a ball. Transfer to the prepared baking sheet. Repeat with the remaining cheese and dough, placing the dough balls ½cm apart on the baking sheet – they should be just touching after proving. Cover with a clean tea towel and leave somewhere warm to rise for 30 mins.

STEP 3

Meanwhile, make the garlic butter. Melt the butter in a small pan over a low heat, then stir in the garlic and rosemary. Remove from the heat and set aside until needed. Heat the oven to 180C/160C fan/gas 4. Brush the risen dough balls with the garlic butter, then bake for 25-30 mins until the dough balls are cooked through and the middles are oozing.

STEP 4

While the dough balls are baking, make the tomato sauce dip. Heat the oil in a saucepan and fry the garlic for 30 seconds. Tip in the passata, vinegar, sugar and chilli flakes, and simmer for 10 mins until thickened. Season to taste and stir in the basil. Brush the warm dough balls with any remaining garlic butter, then serve with the tomato sauce dip on the side for dunking.

Glamorous fairy cakes

Ingredients

For the cakes

140g butter, very well softened

140g golden caster sugar

3 medium eggs

100g self-raising flour

25g custard powder or cornflour

For decorating

600g icing sugar, sifted

6 tbsp water, or half water and half lemon juice, strained

edible green and pink food colourings

crystallised violets

crystallised roses or rose petals

edible wafer flowers

Directions

STEP 1

Heat the oven to 190C/fan 170C/gas 5. Arrange paper cases in bun tins. Put all the cake Ingredients in a large bowl and beat for about 2 mins until smooth. Divide the mixture between the cases so they are half filled and bake for 12-15 mins, until risen and golden. Cool on a wire rack.

STEP 2

Mix the icing sugar and water until smooth and use a third on eight of the cakes. Divide the rest in half, and colour one half pale green and the other half pale pink. Decorate the white ones with crystallised violets, the pink ones with the roses and the green ones with the wafer flowers. Leave to set. Will keep for up to 2-3 days stored in an airtight container in a cool place.

Easy plum jam

Ingredients

2kg plums, stoned and roughly chopped

2kg white granulated sugar

2 tsp ground cinnamon

1 tbsp lemon juice

3 cinnamon sticks (optional)

knob of butter

Directions

STEP 1

Sterilise the jars and any other equipment before you start (see tip). Put a couple of saucers in the freezer, as you'll need these for testing whether the jam is ready later (or use a sugar thermometer). Put the plums in a preserving pan and add 200ml water. Bring to a simmer, and cook for about 10 mins until the plums are tender but not falling apart. Add the sugar, ground cinnamon and lemon juice, then let the sugar dissolve slowly, without boiling. This will take about 10 mins.

STEP 2

Increase the heat and bring the jam to a full rolling boil. After about 5 mins, spoon a little jam onto a cold saucer. Wait a few seconds, then push the jam with your fingertip. If it wrinkles, the jam is ready. If not, cook for a few mins more and test again, with another cold saucer. If you have a sugar thermometer, it will read 105C when ready.

STEP 3

Take the jam off the heat and add the cinnamon sticks (if using) and the knob of butter. The cinnamon will look pretty in the jars and the butter will disperse any scum. Let the jam cool for 15 mins, which will prevent the lumps of fruit sinking to the bottom of the jars. Ladle into hot jars, seal and leave to cool. Will keep for 1 year in a cool, dark place. Chill once opened.

Freezer biscuits

Ingredients

200g pack butter, softened

200g soft brown sugar

2 eggs

1 tsp vanilla extract

200g self-raising flour

140g oats

Your choice of flavours

50g chopped nuts such as pecan, hazelnuts or almonds

50g desiccated coconut

50g raisin, or mixed fruit

Directions

STEP 1

When the butter is really soft, tip it into a bowl along with the sugar. Using an electric hand whisk or exercising some arm muscle, beat together until the sugar is mixed through. Beat in the eggs, one at a time, followed by the vanilla extract and a pinch of salt, if you like. Stir in the flour and oats. The mixture will be quite stiff at this point. Now decide what else you would like to add – any or all of the flavours are delicious – and stir through.

STEP 2

Tear off an A4-size sheet of greaseproof paper. Pile up half the mixture in the middle of the sheet, then use a spoon to thickly spread the mixture along the centre of the paper. Pull over one edge of paper and roll up until you get a tight cylinder. If you have problems getting it smooth, then roll as you would a rolling pin along a kitchen surface. You'll need it to be about the width of a teacup. When it is tightly wrapped, twist up the ends and then place in the freezer. Can be frozen for up to 3 months.

STEP 3

To cook, heat oven to 180C/fan 160C/gas 4 and unwrap the frozen biscuit mix. Using a sharp knife, cut off a disk about ½cm wide. If you have difficulty slicing through, dip the knife into a cup of hot water. Cut off as many biscuits as you need, then pop the mix back into the freezer for another time. Place on a baking sheet, spacing them widely apart as the mixture will spread when cooking, then cook for 15 mins until the tops are golden brown. Leave to cool for at least 5 mins before eating.

Instant berry banana slush

Ingredients

2 ripe bananas

200g frozen berry mix (blackberries, raspberries and currants)

Directions

STEP 1

Slice the bananas into a bowl and add the frozen berry mix. Blitz with a stick blender to make a slushy ice and serve straight away in two glasses with spoons.

Caramelised mushroom tartlets

Ingredients

2 tbsp olive oil

1 onion, chopped

1 tbsp golden caster sugar

250g chestnut mushrooms, cleaned and thinly sliced

1 garlic clove, crushed

3-4 tbsp thyme leaves, finely chopped

butter, for spreading

12 slices of thin sliced white sandwich bread

100g grated gruyère or cheddar, for sprinkling

Directions

STEP 1

Heat the oil in a generous frying pan, add the onion and fry over moderate heat for about 7 mins until soft and golden. Stir in the sugar and seasoning, turn up the heat and add the mushrooms. Sizzle for 5 mins until you have driven off any moisture and the mushrooms are golden. Stir in the garlic for a few further mins, until fragrant, then turn off the heat and stir in most of the thyme (save some for sprinkling). The mushroom mix can be chilled at this point.

STEP 2

To make the tartlet bases, cut 7-8cm circles out of the bread using a cookie cutter or glass. Butter one side and stick buttered-side down into a 12-hole tartlet tin. Freeze any leftovers to make breadcrumbs.

STEP 3

When ready to bake, heat oven to 220C/200 fan/gas 7. Divide the mushroom mixture between the tartlets and top with a sprinkle of cheese. Don't be too tidy about this – any cheese on the tin will form a lacy edge to the tartlets. Bake for 10-15 mins until golden and bubbling. Sprinkle over the reserved herbs and serve.

Ricotta and basil pizza

Ingredients

1 onion, finely chopped

2 yellow peppers, roughly chopped

1 tsp olive oil

2 x 400g/14oz cans chopped tomatoes

500g bag mixed grain or granary bread mix

plain flour, for dusting

10 cherry tomatoes, halved or whole

250g tub ricotta

a few basil leaves, to serve

Directions

STEP 1

Heat oven to 220C/fan 200C/gas 6. Soften the onion and peppers in the oil in a large pan for a few mins. Pour in the tomatoes, season, then simmer for 10 mins.

STEP 2

Meanwhile, make up the bread mix according to pack instructions, then bring the dough together and knead a couple of times. Flour a large baking sheet and roll out the dough into a rectangle roughly 25 x 35cm. Bake for 5 mins on a shelf at the top of the oven until firm.

STEP 3

Remove from the oven, spread with the sauce, add the cherry tomatoes, then dollop over spoonfuls of the ricotta. Bake for 10 mins more until the base is golden and crisp. Scatter with basil and serve straight away with a green salad.

Spiced mackerel on toast with beetroot salsa

Ingredients

250g pack beetroot (not in vinegar), diced

1 eating apple, cut into wedges then thinly sliced

1 small red onion, finely sliced

juice ½ lemon

1 tbsp olive oil, plus extra for drizzling

1 tsp cumin seed

small bunch coriander, leaves roughly chopped

For the fish

4 mackerel fillets, halved widthways

1 tsp curry powder

4 slices sourdough bread or ciabatta

Directions

STEP 1

Mix the beetroot, apple, onion, lemon juice, oil, cumin and coriander together, season well, then set aside while you cook the mackerel. Heat the grill to high. Put the fish onto a sheet of foil on the grill rack, sprinkle over the curry powder, drizzle with oil, then season and rub well into the fish.

STEP 2

Grill for 4-5 mins until the skin is crisp and the fillets are cooked through; you won't need to turn the fish over. Toast the bread in a toaster or alongside the fish under the grill, then drizzle with a little olive oil. Top with the salsa and mackerel, then pour over any pan juices and eat straight away.

DELIGHTFUL RECIPES FOR SIDE DISH

Vegan kimchi

Ingredients

2-3 Chinese leaf (2kg prepared weight)

40-60g sea salt (3% of the cabbage weight)

1 tbsp seaweed (I use wakame), lightly rinsed

1 carrot

½ leek

2 spring onions

For the chilli paste

40g onion, chopped

40g garlic (10 cloves), peeled

5g ginger, chopped

1 small pear, cored and chopped

40g Korean chilli flakes (use less if you prefer it milder)

You will also need

a 2-litre sterilised jar

Instructions

STEP 1

Chop the Chinese leaf into bite-size pieces, weighing it until you have 2kg, then wash under running water. Mix the Chinese leaf with the salt and the seaweed in a large bowl. Set aside.

STEP 2

Every now and then, over the course of 3-4 hrs, mix the salted Chinese leaf and seaweed with your hands. (You will start to see liquid being released.) You want to be able to bend the Chinese leaf without breaking the pieces.

STEP 3

Meanwhile, shred the carrot and leek, and chop the spring onions. Set aside. Make the chilli paste by blitzing the onion, garlic, ginger and pear in a food processor until puréed. Add the chilli flakes, then blitz again to combine. Drain the Chinese leaf mixture, removing as much water as you can. This may take about 10 mins.

STEP 4

Toss the Chinese leaf mixture with the other vegetables, then mix in the chilli paste to coat everything. Tip into a 2-litre sterilised jar. Try not to have too many air pockets and leave a 1-inch space under the lid. Put a fermentation weight on top, or if you don't have one, try using some baking beans in a bag. Keep a plate under the jar in case of overflow. After 24-48 hrs you will begin to see bubbles appearing. That means fermentation is underway.

STEP 5

At any point during the fermentation, you can taste the kimchi to see how you like the flavour. I prefer to keep mine in the fridge after day 3 to slow down the process and start enjoying it. You can transfer the kimchi into smaller jars for easy access from the fridge. It also makes a great present for family and friends.

Gluten-free bread

Ingredients

400g gluten-free white bread flour

1 tsp salt

7g sachet fast-action dried yeast

284ml buttermilk (or the same amount of whole milk with a squeeze of lemon juice)

2 eggs

2 tbsp olive oil

Instructions

STEP 1

Heat oven to 180C/160C fan/gas 4. Mix the flour, salt and yeast in a large bowl. In a separate bowl, whisk together the buttermilk, eggs and oil. Mix the wet ingredients into the dry to make a sticky dough.

STEP 2

Grease a 900g loaf tin, or flour a baking sheet. With oiled hands, shape the dough into a sausage shape for a loaf or a ball for a cob. If making a loaf, place the dough in the tin. For a cob, place it on the baking sheet and score the top with a sharp knife. Cover loosely with a piece of oiled cling film and leave somewhere warm for 1 hr, or until risen by a third or so.

STEP 3

Bake for 50-60 mins until golden and well risen. Turn out onto a wire rack and leave to cool for at least 20 mins before cutting.

Crunchy chopped salad

Ingredients

1 lemon

4 tbsp extra virgin olive oil

1 tsp Dijon mustard

1 tsp honey

10 cherry tomatoes (use a mixture of different colours, if you like)

½ cucumber

2 Little Gem lettuces

1 punnet of cress

100g pomegranate seeds

25g mixed seeds (we used sunflower and pumpkin seeds; see tip below)

You'll also need

chopping board

tea towel or kitchen paper (optional)

sharp knife

citrus juicer

tablespoon

teaspoon

jam jar or small bowl

large salad bowl

kitchen scissors

measuring scales

Instructions

STEP 1

Before you get started take a look at our chopping and knife skills guide. If your chopping board doesn't have anti-slip grips, lay a dampened tea towel or sheet of kitchen paper on the work surface, then place the board on top to stop it from slipping.

STEP 2

Holding the lemon with your hand in the bridge position, cut the lemon in half. Push one half onto a citrus juicer, twist and squeeze to release the juice. Repeat with the second lemon half. Pour the juice into a jam jar or small bowl along with the oil.

STEP 3

Add the mustard, honey and a good pinch each of salt and black pepper. Seal the jar and shake to combine, or whisk the Ingredients together. Will keep covered in the fridge for up to a week.

STEP 4

Cut the tomatoes in half by pinching each one between your thumb and a finger and carefully slicing through the middle with a small serrated knife. Cut each piece in half again to make quarters, then tip the tomatoes into a large bowl.

STEP 5

Wipe down the chopping board, then cut the cucumber in half lengthways. Put the two halves cut-side down on the board so they don't roll around, then cut in half again along the length, so you have four chunky sticks of cucumber. Cut across the cucumber now to make little triangles, keeping your free hand in the claw position with your fingers tucked away from the blade of the knife. Tip the cucumber into the bowl with the tomatoes.

STEP 6

Cut the hard stalk off the lettuces, then cut each lettuce in half and in half again to get four wedges. Working with one lettuce wedge at a time, hold the wedge with your hand in the claw position and chop it into small ribbons – the smaller, the better for this salad. Repeat with the remaining wedges and tip the lettuce into the bowl.

STEP 7

Snip the cress straight into the bowl using kitchen scissors. Weigh out the pomegranate seeds using the scales and add these to the bowl. Repeat with the mixed seeds. Drizzle over roughly half of the dressing over the salad (you will have some leftover) and toss everything together to coat.

Easy onion bhajis

Ingredients

2 onions, finely sliced

100g gram flour

½ tsp gluten-free baking powder

½ tsp chilli powder

½ tsp turmeric

1 green chilli, deseeded and very finely chopped

vegetable oil for frying

For the raita

½ cucumber

150g tub Greek-style yogurt

2 tbsp chopped mint

Instructions

STEP 1

Soak the onion in cold water while you make the base mix. Sift the flour and baking powder into a bowl, then add the chilli powder, turmeric, chopped chilli and a good sprinkling of salt. Mix in about 100ml of cold water to make a thick batter – add a splash more if it feels too stiff.

STEP 2

For the raita, peel the cucumber and grate it into a sieve set over another bowl. Mix the remaining Ingredients with some seasoning and the drained cucumber – squeezing out any extra moisture with your hands – then spoon into a small serving bowl.

STEP 3

Drain the onion well and mix it into the batter. Heat about 5cm of oil in a wok or deep pan. Do not fill the pan more than a third full. Add a tiny speck of batter. If it rises to the surface surrounded by bubbles and starts to brown, then the oil is hot enough for frying.

STEP 4

Lower heaped tbsps of the bhaji mixture into the pan, a few at a time, and cook for a few mins, turning once, until they are evenly browned and crisp, so about 3-4 mins. Drain on kitchen paper, sprinkle with a little salt and keep warm while you cook the rest. Serve with the raita.

cauliflower rice

Ingredients

1 medium cauliflower

good handful coriander, chopped

cumin seeds, toasted (optional)

Instructions

STEP 1

Cut the hard core and stalks from the cauliflower and pulse the rest in a food processor to make grains the size of rice. Tip into a heatproof bowl, cover with cling film, then pierce and microwave for 7 mins on high – there is no need to add any water. Stir in the coriander. For spicier rice, add some toasted cumin seeds.

Polenta bruschetta with tapenade

Ingredients

700ml vegetable stock (Marigold Swiss vegetable bouillon is gluten and dairy-free)

140g instant polenta

2 tbsp chopped fresh basil

2 tbsp olive oil

9 tsp (about half a 190g jar) olive tapenade

9 SunBlush or semi-dried tomatoes, halved

100g mixed salad leaves

Instructions

STEP 1

Bring the stock to the boil in a saucepan, then reduce to a simmer. Stirring continuously, pour in the polenta in a steady steam and cook for 5 mins until thickened. Stir in the basil and season with black pepper and salt, if you like. Spread on an oiled shallow tin measuring 24 x 18cm. Leave to set for 1 hr.

STEP 2

Cut the polenta into 9 rectangles, each 8 x 6cm, then cut in half diagonally to make triangle shapes. Heat a griddle until hot, brush each triangle with oil and grill for 4-5 mins each side, until crisp and golden.

STEP 3

Top each triangle with ½ tsp tapenade and half a tomato. Serve warm on salad leaves.

Hasselback potatoes

Ingredients

1.5kg medium-sized floury potatoes (Maris piper or King Edward work well), peeled if you like

4 tbsp vegetable oil

4 garlic cloves, bashed

a few sprigs of rosemary

sea salt flakes

Instructions

STEP 1

Heat the oven to 200C/180C fan/gas 6. Use a metal skewer and insert through the back of one of the flatter sides of the potato. It should go through most of the potato. Place on a chopping board, skewer-side down, and slice through the potato (be careful not to cut all the way through on both ends). You can also put each potato in-between two handles of wooden spoons, and cut through to the spoon, if this is easier for you. A sharp knife will help to make slices a few mm apart. Remove the skewer and repeat with the remaining potatoes.

STEP 2

Put the potatoes cut-side up on a shallow baking tray and drizzle over the oil. Rub each potato with your hands to coat well in the oil, getting some in between the slices. Toss in the bashed garlic, rosemary, and season well. Roast for 50 mins – 1 hr until the potatoes are tender throughout and the tops are golden and crisp. Baste with any oil in the pan halfway cooking to get extra crisp potatoes.

Brown rice tabbouleh with eggs & parsley

Ingredients

75g brown basmati rice

fresh thyme, a sprig

160g celery, chopped

2 large eggs

1 tsp vegetable bouillon

1 small lemon, zest and juice

1 small red onion, finely chopped

3 tbsp parsley, chopped

1/2 pomegranate, seeds only

Instructions

STEP 1

Simmer the rice with the thyme and celery for 20 mins until tender. Meanwhile, boil the eggs for 7 mins, then cool in cold water and carefully peel off the shell.

STEP 2

Drain the rice and tip into a bowl. Add the bouillon, lemon zest and juice, and red onion, then stir well and scatter over the parsley and pomegranate. Spoon onto plates or into lunchboxes, then halve or quarter the eggs and arrange on top.

Crispy Jerusalem artichokes with roasted garlic & rosemary

Ingredients

800g Jerusalem artichokes

1 garlic bulb, cut down the middle

1 tbsp rosemary leaves, chopped

3 tbsp rapeseed oil

pinch ground mace

20g butter

2 tsp lemon juice

Instructions

STEP 1

Heat oven to 180C/160C fan/gas 4. Soak the artichokes in cold water for 20 mins or so to loosen any dirt, then scrub them with a scourer, being sure to remove any grit. Halve the small ones and quarter the bigger ones, and put them in a roasting tin with the split garlic bulb and rosemary. Coat everything with the oil and season. Roast for 45-50 mins until tender inside and crispy outside.

STEP 2

To finish, squeeze the softened garlic cloves from their skins and toss with the roasted artichokes, along with the mace, butter and lemon juice.

Spiced apple crisps

Ingredients

2 Granny Smiths

cinnamon, for sprinkling

Instructions

STEP 1

Heat the oven to 160C/ 140C fan/ gas mark 3. Core the apple and slice through the equator into very thin slices 1 - 2mm thick. Dust with cinnamon and lay flat on a baking sheet lined with parchment paper.

STEP 2

Cook for 45 mins – 1 hour, turning halfway through and removing any crisps that have turned brown. Continue cooking until the apples have dried out and are light golden. Cool, store in an airtight container and enjoy as a snack.

Quick pickled cucumbers

Ingredients

1 large cucumber, ends trimmed, cut in half widthways and spiralized into thick ribbons

1 tsp flaky sea salt

1 tbsp white wine vinegar

1 tbsp caster sugar

½ tsp coriander seeds

a small handful of dill, leaves picked

Instructions

STEP 1

Toss the cucumber ribbons with the salt in a colander. Leave for 15 mins then squeeze out any excess moisture with your hands and pat the ribbons dry with a tea towel.

STEP 2

Mix the other ingredients together in a small bowl then stir in the cucumber.

Air-fryer brussels sprouts

Ingredients

350g fresh brussels sprouts, or 250g frozen

1 tsp vegetable oil

chopped cooked bacon, chilli flakes or chopped roasted hazelnuts, to serve (optional)

Instructions

STEP 1

Heat the air fryer to 180C. If using fresh sprouts, trim them, then tip in a bowl. Drizzle over the oil, season well and toss to coat. Arrange the sprouts in the air-fryer basket in a single layer and cook for 10-15, tossing halfway through.

STEP 2

If cooking from frozen, tip the frozen sprouts into the air-fryer basket and cook for 10-15 mins, depending on how golden you like them. Remove, then tip onto a serving plate and scatter with any of the suggested toppings, if you like.

Malabar prawns

Ingredients

400g raw king prawns

2 tsp turmeric

3-4 tsp Kashmiri chilli powder

4 tsp lemon juice, plus a squeeze

40g ginger, half peeled and grated, half finely sliced into matchsticks

1 tbsp vegetable oil

4 curry leaves

2-4 green chillies, halved and deseeded

1 onion, finely sliced

1 tsp cracked black pepper

40g fresh coconut, grated

½ small bunch coriander, leaves only

Instructions

STEP 1

Rinse the prawns in cold water and pat dry. Toss them with the turmeric, chilli powder, lemon juice and grated ginger and set aside.

STEP 2

Heat the oil in a pan and add the curry leaves, chilli, sliced ginger and onion. Cook until translucent, about 10 mins, then add the black pepper.

STEP 3

Toss the prawns in with any marinade, and stir-fry until cooked, about 2 mins. Season if required and add a squeeze of lemon juice. Serve sprinkled with the coconut and coriander leaves.

Pickled red onions

Ingredients

300ml cider vinegar

3 tbsp golden caster sugar

1 tbsp sea salt flakes

6 black peppercorns

6 coriander seeds

1 star anise

1 bay leaf

3 small red onions, sliced into rings

Instructions

STEP 1

Pour the vinegar into a pan, add the sugar, sea salt, the spices and bay leaf, and bring to a simmer. After

1 min, check that the sugar and salt have dissolved. Remove from the heat.

STEP 2

Boil the kettle. Put the onion slices in a sieve or colander. Pour over the hot water from the kettle and drain well. When cool enough to handle, pack the onion rings into a 500g sterilised jar. Pour over the warm vinegar and seal. Cool, then chill and leave to pickle for 2 hrs. Will keep for 6 months unopened, or 2 weeks in the fridge once opened.

5
TO WRAP THINGS UP!

You can take steps – in addition to medication – to help manage your symptoms:

Exercise: You can strengthen muscles around your affected joints with gentle exercise. It also may improve your fatigue. Check with your doctor before you start a workout program. Don't put stress on joints that are tender. Low-impact exercises to try include swimming, walking, cycling, and water aerobics.

Heat and ice: When you apply heat to an affected joint, it can ease pain and relax stiff muscles. When you apply cold to your joint, the numbing effect can dull your pain. Cold also can reduce swelling.

Relaxation: Techniques such as breathing exercises and guided imagery can help reduce your stress and may help ease pain.

Sleep: You need your rest to help your body cope with RA. Limit caffeine late in the day, stay off electronic devices before bedtime, and make sure you take your medicine on schedule.

Education: Programs that teach self-management skills for people with chronic diseases can improve your quality of life. Ask your doctor for information about local programs.

Rheumatoid arthritis diet

Changing what you eat may help with your RA symptoms. Adding healthy fats, and avoiding unhealthy fats and processed foods high in carbohydrates, can help reduce inflammation. You might also lose weight, which can ease stress on your joints. If you have RA, you're at higher risk of cardiovascular disease. Moving toward a heart-healthy diet can reduce your chances of heart disease.

Takeaways

Rheumatoid arthritis is an autoimmune disorder that can affect your joints as well as other parts of your body. When you have it, your joints become swollen, painful, and stiff. There's no cure for RA, but treatments can help relieve your symptoms. Lifestyle changes, such as altering your diet, getting plenty of rest, and low-impact exercise, also may ease the effects of RA.

www.ingramcontent.com/pod-product-compliance
Lightning Source LLC
Chambersburg PA
CBHW071826210526
45479CB00001B/18